D1264211

The Rise and Fall of the Biopsychosocial Model

Reconciling Art and Science in Psychiatry

S. Nassir Ghaemi, M.D., M.P.H.
Professor, Department of Psychiatry
Tufts University School of Medicine
Boston, Massachusetts

The Johns Hopkins University Press
Baltimore

© 2010 The Johns Hopkins University Press
All rights reserved. Published 2010
Printed in the United States of America on acid-free paper
9 8 7 6 5 4 3 2 1

The Johns Hopkins University Press
2715 North Charles Street
Baltimore, Maryland 21218-4363
www.press.jhu.edu

Library of Congress Cataloging-in-Publication Data

Ghaemi, S. Nassir.
    The rise and fall of the biopsychosocial model : reconciling art
and science in psychology / S. Nassir Ghaemi.
        p. ; cm.
    Includes bibliographical references and index.
    ISBN-13: 978-0-8018-9390-2 (hardcover : alk. paper)
    ISBN-10: 0-8018-9390-9 (hardcover : alk. paper)
    1. Eclectic psychotherapy. 2. Biological psychiatry. 3. Social psychiatry.
I. Title.
    [DNLM: 1. Psychiatry—methods. 2. Mental Disorders—therapy.
3. Models, Biological. 4. Models, Psychological. 5. Psychological Theory.
WM 100 G411r 2009]
    RC489.E24G43 2009
    616.89′14-dc22   2009009808

A catalog record for this book is available from the British Library.

Special discounts are available for bulk purchases of this book.
For more information, please contact Special Sales at 410-516-6936
or specialsales@press.jhu.edu.

The Johns Hopkins University Press uses environmentally friendly
book materials, including recycled text paper that is composed of at least
30 percent post-consumer waste, whenever possible. All of our book papers
are acid-free, and our jackets and covers are printed on paper with
recycled content.

For Leston Havens, who made me think and *feel,*
and in memory of Paul Roazen, intellectual honesty personified

For each of the great problems of life, there is a solution: simple, plausible, and wrong.   H. L. MENCKEN

Contents

Preface

Half a century ago, John Kenneth Galbraith developed the concept of *conventional wisdom* to denote how we often seek acceptability, rather than truth, in our theories (Galbraith 1958). In psychiatry, conventional wisdom today is the biopsychosocial model. It is highly accepted and is generally viewed as innocuous, yet whether this is true is questioned all too infrequently.

I have doubts about the biopsychosocial model. If not untrue, it has at least far outrun the purposes it originally served. Psychiatry is currently eclectic, verging on anarchic. For all the advances in neurobiology and psychopharmacology and for all the expertise in psychotherapies, the field has no overarching conceptual structure. Or, perhaps better said, what passes for a conceptual schema for the field—the biopsychosocial model—rose from the ashes of psychoanalysis and is dying on the shoals of neurobiology.

The current unpalatable psychiatric status quo is not too different from the view decades ago of prominent American psychiatrist, Roy Grinker, the underrecognized founder of psychiatry's biopsychosocial model (Grinker 1970, p. 730): "Modern psychiatry has been extended as a total field as broad as life, giving more and more room for its mad ride in all directions. Some psychiatric groups attempt to overcome this manic phase by fencing off a limited space—the isolation of schools and ideologies. Others, as eclectics, wander aimlessly over the entire pasture. A more common solution, persisting through the ages, has been to assume either a reductionistic or a humanistic position with some lip service to the other."

The biopsychosocial eclecticism prescribed by Grinker and others has both anesthetized and destabilized this profession. On the one hand, some are discontented and disoriented; many practitioners as well as the people they treat are confused about what psychiatry is all about: is it primarily biological, or mostly psychotherapeutic, or a mix? And, if a mix, what is it a mixture of? The biopsychosocial model pretends to answer these questions, though unsatisfactorily. On the other hand, many in the field are complacent. Biopsychosocial eclecticism is broad and benign enough to make everyone feel accepted. Any theory can work and any perspective can fit; hence, there is little impetus for many to question their own theories or perspectives. Yet before one can seek new answers, one has to become uncomfortable with past answers. Before we can move ahead and take the next step in approximating what is true, we need to be convinced that change is necessary.

When I presented this material to a department of psychiatry that had been highly devoted to the biopsychosocial model for decades, one of the critiques I received was that my analysis was purely negative. I did not provide a better alternative to the biopsychosocial model, while I admitted that it was an advance over previous dogmatisms. While you work on a better theory, my colleagues advised me, leave us our biopsychosocial model for now, with all its faults.

Indeed, a negative critique only paves the way for a better alternative; as George Washington once reputedly said, people must feel before they can see. Mental health professionals and the public must come to realize that there is something deeply wrong with the status quo before they will be open to alternatives. The point of this book is to make the reader uneasy, to demonstrate the inadequacy of the biopsychosocial model, and to show that it now needs to be superseded.

As to what should replace it, I think it needs to be a model that is both nondogmatic and noneclectic. I have tried to describe that alternative in more detail separately, and in part III I expand on it. The main problem, though, is not the absence of alternatives; the main problem is lack of awareness that there is a problem.

I am convinced now that many in psychiatry and other mental health professions will not listen to any alternative models because they are too comfortable with their assumptions. For them, Galbraith's other dictum applies: "If you cannot comfort the afflicted, you can at least afflict the comfortable."

Perhaps it is time to afflict the comfortable.

Acknowledgments

This book is a sequel to *The Concepts of Psychiatry,* seeking to provide a rationale for why the positive program set forward in that book should be taken seriously. Thus, it shares many of the same debts and acknowledgments of that earlier work, to which I must add and repeat a few. Any writer is in debt to his family's tolerance for the solitary work of writing, and—despite having delayed this project after the birth of my son, Zane, in 2003, until the end of his second year—I am no exception. No person has had more influence on me personally or intellectually than has my father, Kamal Ghaemi, M.D.

   Rudolph Makkreel, at Emory University, a philosopher with expertise in the work of Wilhelm Dilthey, was generous with his time and helpful in revision of sections of the book. Howard Kushner, of the Emory School of Public Health, helped me think through how to understand work in the history of psychiatry. Ronald Pies provided comments on the sections written about the humanities, as did Gareth Owen on selected chapters. The bulk of the manuscript of this book was presented to a gathered conference of the Department of Psychiatry at the Johns Hopkins University in January 2008. I thank the department for its attentiveness to these ideas and the helpful feedback I received from its faculty and staff, in particular current chairman Raymond DePaulo and past chairman Paul McHugh. Phillip Slavney deserves special thanks for extensive discussion of these themes and his suggestion that I delve more deeply into *Verstehen*.

Versions of the book were also presented in numerous conference settings, leading to valuable feedback that helped guide the book along its way. Those who heard these ideas and helped me think about them include the audience at a symposium of the American Psychiatric Association annual meeting and the departments of psychiatry of Northwestern, Case Western, and Yale Universities, the Cleveland Clinic, and the Universities of Tehran, Chile, and São Paolo. At Northwestern, I especially benefited from meeting and learning from Sidney Weissman, a former pupil of Roy Grinker, who introduced me to the relevance of Grinker's ideas at a point in the manuscript where I had not come across his work. Toward the end, I debated the book's main themes with the local Boston chapter of the Association for the Advancement of Philosophy and Psychiatry, led by Jennifer Radden; the gentle peer review of one's friends is invaluable. I also thank Brett Mulder, a psychology graduate student, for thinking through my ideas about *Verstehen* with me. The appreciation I express for the input of my friends and colleagues is not meant to imply their assent to some, or even most, of the ideas I express here.

Wendy Harris has remained a supportive and helpful editor at the Johns Hopkins University Press, and I thank her and her staff for all their efforts. Major portions of this book were written in the bohemian but welcoming confines of Aurora Coffeehouse, in the Virginia Highlands neighborhood of Atlanta, Georgia; if I could also thank the coffee that kept me going, I would.

Leston Havens has been the most formative intellectual influence I have had among psychiatrists. He also introduced me to the late Paul Roazen. Paul was a man whom I knew from his books and whom I grew to love as a man. He passed away suddenly, and I have felt the void ever since. After our wonderful conversations (and after reading his books even more intensely), I realize what a pioneer he was and how forthright he had always been about seeking the truth, despite personal or professional cost, a characteristic that most of us do not possess. I tried in this book to live up to his standard of intellectual honesty.

Part I / The Rise of the Biopsychosocial Model

CHAPTER ONE

The Perils of Open-mindedness

Adolf Meyer's Psychobiology

The story of psychiatry is usually told as a battle between two dogmas: those who see mental illness as simply a brain disease and those who view psychoanalysis as the ultimate solution. This simplified analysis explains much: nineteenth-century European psychiatry was predominantly biological and twentieth-century American psychiatry was mostly psychoanalytic, and now the pendulum is swinging back in the biological direction, at least as far as treating major mental illnesses is concerned.

But the story of this battle does not explain the dilemmas of psychiatry today. For even though psychopharmacology is so predominant in treating certain conditions, we live in an eclectic era, a time when all theories are possible, and all perspectives are valued—and yet no sense is made of it all. Our eclectic psychiatry is a flawed attempt at solving the conflict between the two dogmas, a failure that began in the early twentieth century, when a diminutive, goateed Swiss immigrant took over the most prestigious psychiatric post in the United States. When Adolf Meyer became the chair of psychiatry at the Johns Hopkins University, he brought with him not only a classical training in nineteenth-century Germanic psychiatry but also a firm resolve to enact the ideas of American pragmatism. By this I mean not only the practical how-to attitudes of American culture but also the formal philosophy of pragmatism, which Meyer had learned at the feet of its leading advocate, John Dewey (Meyer 1948, p. 152). The result was Meyer's "psychobiology" (Meyer 1948), a precursor of today's biopsychosocial (BPS) model.

But Meyer was not only the chair at Johns Hopkins; he was the president of the American Psychiatric Association. As such, he was the leader of the field of psychiatry in the first half of the twentieth century. Meyer ultimately failed as a leader, and his eclectic approach continues to fail today, because, when the profession needed a democratic leader, one who guided without tyrannizing, it got nothing but anarchy. The reasons for drawing this conclusion are based on a story that begins with Meyer a hundred years ago and ends where we are today.

The Rejection of Disease

The first important aspect of Meyer's approach was that he opposed the concepts of disease and syndrome, such as those used by Emil Kraepelin (the main leader of nineteenth-century German biological psychiatry). Meyer proposed viewing psychiatric conditions as "reactions" to life events. His psychobiology was meant to incorporate the importance of biology, while subordinating it to the individual person.

> We study behavior not merely as a function of the mind and of various parts of the body, but as a function of the individual, and by that we mean the living organism, not a mysteriously split entity. When we see somebody eating or drinking too much or too hurriedly, or overworking, with inadequate recreation, we want to know why and how this occurs, and we modify it not merely as a state of mind but as behavior. That is what we imply by psychobiological—undivided and direct attention to the person and to the function, health, and efficiency of the person as a living organism. . . . We study the facts (a fact is anything which makes a difference) for what they mean in actual life, and by that we mean the life of a "somebody." He is to us an organism with a life history, a biography. (Meyer 1948, pp. 434–36)

In practice, Meyer's psychobiology was hostile toward biological approaches: one could not, in the prepsychopharmacology era, change biology. The biological component of mental illness was seen as equivalent to genetics, and hereditary constitution was inherently unchangeable. Being a pragmatist, Meyer wanted to focus on what would produce results—biology was a dead end. Thus, Meyer's psychobiology was a psychosociology of mental illness. In Meyer's own hands, this approach had some benefits: he focused on the social aspects of mental illness, was a founder of the field of psychiatric epidemiology,[1] coined the term *mental hygiene,* and was a key figure in the early advocacy movement of those experiencing mental illness.

Holism

As far as individuals seeking treatment are concerned, the consequence of Meyer's approach was a pragmatic flexibility that, in its negative connotation, involved a willingness to do anything, even if it actually ended up doing harm. Perhaps the best description of his views is provided by one of his students (Muncie 1974, p. 705):

> The psychobiology of Meyer had two assumptions: (1) that the living man can only be studied as a whole person in action, and (2) that this whole person represents an integrat[ion] of hierarchically arranged functions. . . . The fundamental concept of psychobiology is that of integration. According to this concept, man is the indivisible unit of study, but this study can be approached from any of a number of hierarchically arranged levels: the physicochemical, the reflex . . . and the psychobiological, that is, the activity of the whole person, as an item of biography. . . . Briefly, the whole is greater than the sum of the parts. The activity at any level may be altered by change at either a higher or a lower level.

These views of Meyer can later be clearly seen in the works of the founders of the biopsychosocial model—Roy Grinker and George Engel (chapters 3 and 4). Treatment involved an appreciation of the whole person from a longitudinal view of the entire life history, not just in a cross-sectional assessment of the present: "Treatment may be instituted at any level of integration which can be shown to be involved in the origin of disorder. This leads to multiple attacks on the most diverse problems in treatment, for example (a) simple psychotherapy as well as chemical attack on bromide delirium or (b) electroshock treatment as well as psychotherapy in depression" (p. 706).

Meyer's view also prefigured the field of psychosomatic medicine, which would later spawn the BPS model, as well as the view that a similar model should apply to all of medicine:

> Meyer often remarked that there seemed to be but a few ways in which people could react. This underscores the clinical fact that the diversity of life experience

must finally be channeled into a few varieties of behavioral expression. . . . The emphasis in psychobiology . . . has been on the effort to elucidate the interrelations of life experience . . . and their biological means of expression. Actually, this means an effort at synthesis of the statistically valid descriptive generalities of mental disease (form) and the dynamic aspects (content) imparting meaning (that is, plausibility). This is that search which "psychosomatic medicine" has appropriated peculiarly to itself but which applies in all psychiatry if, indeed, not in all medicine. (Muncie 1974)

Treatment as Negotiation

Meyer's disciple noted that the thinker was not particularly detailed in his treatment guidance:

In rereading Meyer's contributions to psychiatry one is struck by the few discussions of detailed treatment methods. The most vivid memory I have of his attitude to treatment does not appear in his collected works but derives from a statement made in a staff meeting late in his tenure at the Phipps Psychiatric Clinic. . . . "The patient comes with his own view of his trouble; the physician has another view. Treatment consists of the joint effort to bring about that approximation of those views which will be the most effective and the most satisfying in the situation." This struck me forcibly at the time, for it laid down what I recognized had been our established working method at the clinic. . . . This succinctly asserts a cardinal principle: Treatment is a matter of negotiation of viewpoints and attitudes. This discards immediately old authoritarian views of treatment. (Muncie 1974)

He goes on to explain that the individual seeking treatment is the ultimate source of decision, and the physician, except in rare cases of clear danger, needs to try to convince the individual about the best course of action, while constantly being open to the person's preferences. While this respect for autonomy is laudable, and this pragmatic recognition of the role of the values of the patient and the physician is important, there is a flip side to the Meyerian approach: *little is ever insisted on.*

The author identifies Meyer's values-based, deeply eclectic, interpretation of pragmatism: "For him the psychiatrist was a negotiator, working with the raw material of observable malfunction, with the purpose of assisting in the creation of a meaningful (that is, acceptably plausible) history up to the present; and from that creation the opening of new and better (that is, less threatening and more fulfilling and rewarding) options for the future. This goal is not unlike the creative artist's and avails itself of the most diverse theoretical views and methods. Always comes the ultimate test: Does it work?" (Muncie 1974).

A final prediction is made: "Much of current theory and practice must be looked on as dispensable at a date not to far distant. If I were to be asked what of the Meyerian tradition will likely live, I would single out the integration concept and treatment as negotiation." In fact, much more of the Meyerian tradition is alive and well today, covertly so, because it has been reconceptualized, for better or for worse, as the biopsychosocial model.

Meyer and Biological Radicals

Meyer's approach to treatment as negotiation stemmed from his eclectic attitude: congenial personally, he seemed congenitally incapable of disagreeing with any person. Any idea, even the most hare-brained, would receive a respectful hearing from Meyer. While quaint and commendable pedagogically, this excessive open-mindedness left American psychiatry—so dependent on Meyer's opinions—open to the influence of more hard-headed biological radicals and psychoanalytic dogmatists.

The Colectomy Cure

It is underappreciated, for instance, that Meyer played a key role in legitimizing two particularly extreme biological approaches. The first, developed by Henry Cotton, was the focal toxin theory of mental illness; the idea that mental illness was caused by toxins released by bacteria in the body, the specific locations of which were the colon and rotted teeth. Sure enough, Cotton observed that many patients with mental illness had rotten teeth; by pulling those teeth, he observed improvement in many patients with psychosis. If rotten teeth were not observed, patients underwent abdominal surgery, at which time large focal infectious swellings would be observed in the colon. Colonic resection would then lead to improvement. Cotton's methods consisted of a collection of about one hundred case reports, with mostly short-term follow-up, published in his prominent text, *The Defective Delinquent and Insane* (Cotton 1921), which Meyer legitimized by writing a generous foreword. In the 1920s, one cannot fault Cotton or Meyer for using poor clinical research methods (e.g., randomized clinical trials, which would have shown the biases in Cotton's methods, were not used in medical research until 1948). Yet Meyer's authority was powerful enough to render Cotton's work much more credible than it might otherwise have been. In the 1920s to 1930s, tens of thousands of colectomies and full mouth teeth extractions were conducted in patients with mental illness. (Meyer himself sometimes recommended it.)[2] This practice continued until Cotton died and other physicians lost faith in the treatment.

Frontal Lobotomy

The other biological extremist story is more famous (though again Meyer's role is generally underappreciated): psychosurgery. Promoted in the United States by Walter Freeman, the idea was that mental illness reflected abnormal function of the frontal lobes. With frontal lobotomy, the belief was that the disconnection of that part of the brain would lead to diminished mental symptoms, if not an outright cure. Freeman presented the results from his first few cases in a 1936 conference in Baltimore. The concept of surgery on the brain was about as extreme an approach to biological psychiatry as anyone could have imagined. Many psychoanalyst attendees were convinced that mental illness was psychological in origin and had nothing to do with the brain. They protested that Freeman was proposing nothing but mutilation of the brain.

At the conference, Meyer's intervention turned the tide for Freeman: "I am not antagonistic to this work, but find it very interesting," he said; he went on to simply ask for careful and cautious research. "The work should be in the hands of those who are willing and ready to heed the necessary indications for such a responsible step, and to follow up scrupulously the experience with each case. . . . At the hands of Dr. Freeman and Dr. Watts I know these conditions will be lived up to" (El-Hai 2005). As the founder of American eclecticism, Meyer, unfortunately, could not bring any effective critique to bear on dangerous and unproven methods that would soon get out of hand.

Meyer in effect gave Freeman a foothold in mainstream psychiatry, a foothold that Freeman exploited for more than twenty years, with the result that hundreds of thousands of persons received frontal lobotomies. The story was not too different from Cotton. Freeman basically reported many cases observed over certain periods of time. In contrast to Cotton, Freeman observed many cases for long durations, and some credit must be given for those efforts.

Unfortunately, Freeman, like Cotton, was a brain dogmatist, and he became more and more convinced in his own ideology. As a result, he began to use frontal lobotomy more and more extensively, not just as a treatment of last resort in the most ill schizophrenics (as in the first cases presented to Meyer) but later as a treatment of first resort for the mildest mood disorders; not just for "backward schizophrenics," but for unhappy citizens of all ilk (such as Rosemary, the unfortunate daughter of Joseph P. Kennedy, who likely experienced a mood disorder but became intellectually impaired due to her lobotomy). By 1950 Freeman had personally conducted 2,400 transorbital lobotomies, an "office procedure" that allowed him to lobotomize a patient in fifteen minutes (El-Hai 2005).[3]

This ineffective and harmful treatment did not die until its founder died, simultaneous with the rise of antipsychotic medications, which provided a safer alternative to getting severely psychotic patients out of mental asylums.

Meyer as Enabler

Meyer's role was as an *enabler*: Meyer was so eclectic, so open to other ideas, that he could not stand firm against even the harmful ones. One cannot claim that Meyer could not have foreseen the dangers of those treatments; plenty of his contemporaries did. It did not take a huge amount of courage or wisdom to realize that large-scale removal of the colon in persons with mental illness was not justified based on the available scientific evidence as well as the risks. It did not take much knowledge to recognize that frontal lobotomy was a drastic procedure with minimal scientific backing and a high risk of poor outcomes. As famed neurosurgeon Wilder Penfield told Freeman on one occasion, "Walter, don't you realize that you're doing a very dangerous thing?" (El-Hai 2005).

Perhaps Meyer's reaction to these dangerous theories was partly personal. He knew both Cotton and Freeman well: Cotton had been Meyer's student, and Freeman had served with Meyer for about a decade on the newly formed American Board of Psychiatry and Neurology. Perhaps personal comfort led Meyer to trust their scientific integrity more than he should have. A key problem was that both Cotton and Freeman were biological dogmatists, and they did not pursue their theories with the open-mindedness that the eclectic Meyer would have preferred.

The larger problem is that Meyer's eclecticism was unable to provide a rationale to resist Cotton and Freeman. Meyer's psychobiology would argue that such biological approaches should be explored. Despite his own predilection to the contrary, Meyer had no argument why these biological theories should not be pursued. Any theory in principle could be correct. There was no specific reason why one theory would be seen as more effective than another. Why not lobotomize the mildly depressed person?

Ideas have consequences. Eclecticism, even when extreme, as with Meyer, would seem to be benign. Yet given the influence that Meyer and his eclecticism had on

American psychiatry for much of the twentieth century, the possibility exists that Meyer's worldview may be partly responsible for the maiming, and sometimes even the deaths, of those harmed by the biological extremism that flourished under the umbrella of his eclecticism. In politics, according to a Napoleonic maxim, a mistake is not just a mistake; it is treason. Because a politician makes decisions that affect many lives, mistakes can cause death and destruction; hence, politicians need to be held to a higher standard, in this view. Physicians are similarly placed in the moral universe. Meyer's mistakes had ramifications in the lives of the tens of thousands of people who were subjected to these operations and to their loved ones, and a greater responsibility is borne by those mistakes. His eclecticism had sad consequences.

Abetting Psychoanalysis

Meyer's eclecticism, thus, was unable to inoculate psychiatry from biological dogmatism. It also failed to prevent the rise of the proponents of the mind dogma: psychoanalytic orthodoxy. Again, while Meyer himself was more socially oriented and kept psychoanalytic orthodoxy at arm's length, the eclectic approach to psychiatry that he fostered gave plenty of room for the psychoanalytic movement to expand in the United States. By the 1960s, after Meyer's death, psychoanalytic dogmatism was paramount.

Politically, socially, and economically, psychoanalysis exerted almost total control over American psychiatry from the 1940s to the 1980s. In those two generations, it is perhaps not an exaggeration to reflect that legions of bright psychiatrists were, more or less, brainwashed by the mind dogma, and, worse, many mentally ill people were treated with a method that was essentially ineffective for them (e.g., psychoanalysis for schizophrenia was common for decades until proven ineffective in the 1980s). Not as directly harmful as lobotomy or colectomy, widespread psychoanalysis was perhaps more indirectly harmful by sidetracking entire generations of doctors and patients into a dead-end theory.

Psychiatric Anarchist

Adolf Meyer was widely respected during and after his life. He was open-minded, to a fault, and his psychobiology seemed so benign and eclectic that almost no one has ever perceived a reason to criticize it. Yet, Meyer's eclecticism was so extreme that he was unable to provide any real leadership to American psychiatry; on his

watch, doctors and patients were not protected from extreme biological dogmatism (or psychoanalytic hegemony). His thinking was so libertarian, even anar-
chistic, that he could not lead.

A few perceptive mavericks saw that Meyer's eclecticism had left psychiatry un-
rooted, as the field swayed back and forth between biological and psychoanalytic
dogmatism (Grinker 1964a). They determined that something needed to be done.
Perhaps, they thought, Meyer's eclecticism could be improved on. We will now examine these improvements.

CHAPTER TWO

So Many Theories, So Little Time

The Rise of Eclecticism

In 1954, as new president of the Canadian Psychological Association, D. C. Williams gave an incoming address titled "The New Eclecticism" (Williams 1954). In it he identified the key dilemma in psychology as the wars between behaviorism and psychoanalysis—two incompatible theoretical systems. Eclecticism was "a simpleminded, though anything but simplifying, way out of the dilemma." He noted how previously the term *eclectic* had a connotation of contempt, that in the 1950s it was beginning to be rehabilitated, and defined the "new eclecticism" as follows:

> We have, it seems to me, drastically and advantageously shifted our ground. Whereas one previously adopted a theoretical position and argued it from within that frame of reference, now we realize the advantages which may accrue if any number of given positions are found to be approachable from without the particular frame of reference each espouses. It has occurred to many of our number that merely to criticize Theory A from the vantage point of Theory B is unlikely to produce any other effect than a rejoinder in kind and so ad infinitum. . . . It is this current concern to find an alternative, unbiased vantage point from which to view dispassionately the whole field of theory which I term *the new eclecticism*. (D. C. Williams 1954)

He also noted that the new eclecticism would not necessarily lead to a general over-arching theory: "These methodological considerations produce general agreement on the rules of the game rather than general acceptance of a specific theoretical position. They produce, as it were, a *modus vivendi* without cordiality" (D. C. Williams 1954).[1]

Similarly, some psychiatrists (G. M. Abroms 1969) described the "old eclecticism" as being "against orthodoxy but not for anything." In the case of psychology as a discipline, the big conflict at the time was between behaviorism, based on the work of Pavlov and Skinner, and psychoanalysis. Psychologists had to choose between accepting one or the other of those mutually exclusive theories, or becoming eclectic, using both. The old eclecticism was one of theory; the problem was that the theories were incompatible.

By the 1950s and 1960s, the "new eclecticism" was sometimes seen as an eclecticism of method rather than one of theory. Yet even then some critics identified risks, one being the danger that this new eclecticism would "disintegrate into shotgun application of too many techniques for poorly rationalized and inconsistent purposes" (G. M. Abroms 1969). To avoid this outcome, the new eclectics insisted on a "unified field theory," often identified with general systems theory (GST; see chapter 5). In essence, the new eclectics argued that the old orthodoxies could be (and should be) replaced by the new eclecticism if the GST succeeded as a viable overall theoretical framework. Translated into psychiatric language, the biopsychosocial (BPS) model (as the psychiatric equivalent of the GST) was the theoretical basis for the contemporary eclecticism of psychiatry. As an approach, eclecticism stands or falls with the BPS model, which in turn is based on the GST. If either theory fails, then we are faced with the dangers so clearly elucidated by some early critics: "dilettantism, superficiality, dehumanization, and lack of theoretical framework" (G. M. Abroms 1969).[2]

Psychological Studies of Eclecticism

Most psychotherapists view their practice as eclectic (Dimond, Havens, and Jones 1978). In limited empirical research on the topic (Garfield and Kurtz 1977), it appears that eclectic psychotherapists have a similar general philosophy but differ widely in practice. Eclecticism appears to reflect concern for individualization of treatment: "An effort to integrate the ideas, concepts, and techniques of many psychotherapists into a broad framework that permits and facilitates the development of patient-specific treatment strategies. Basic to this approach is an emphasis on the appreciation of each patient as a unique individual who functions in a particular environment" (Dimond, Havens, and Jones 1978).

Of the few empirical studies about the nature of eclecticism in psychology, two used similar methods to study this topic in three different decades (Garfield and Kurtz 1977; Dimond, Havens, and Jones 1978; Norcross, Karpiak, and Lister 2005). In all three decades, the largest single self-identification by psychotherapists was as eclectic or "integrative," the latter defined as seeking to put together many methods in a single whole. In 1977, most psychotherapists mixed psychoanalytic and learning theory methods; in 1988 and again in 2005, they mixed cognitive methods with behavioral, humanistic, or psychoanalytic approaches. Despite the mixing of methods, the core method shifted from psychoanalysis in the 1970s to cognitive therapy currently. Why the change? One might argue that some growth in empirical research has favored cognitive therapy; others might argue the influence of fads and more subjective factors; most likely both are relevant.

In 2005, when asked about what they meant by integration or eclecticism, 85 percent of psychiatrists endorsed the concept of a *broader* theoretical orientation than specific schools, rather than the *absence* of a theoretical orientation. Again, we see that eclecticism and a broad theory, like the BPS model, go hand-in-hand. Also, when asked about the concept of broad theoretical integration as opposed to the notion of technical eclecticism (using specific methods as opposed to paying attention to their underlying theories), most therapists preferred the former, suggesting an evolution away from the early technical eclecticism of the 1950s and 1960s.

When asked to explain their eclectic views, the most common definition provided by therapists (representing 34% to 47% of responses in 1977, 1988, and 2005) was along the lines of the following: "Use whatever theory or method seems best for the client. Select procedures according to the client and/or problem." The next most common response was: "Use and combine two or three theories in therapy," followed by "amalgamation of theories or aspects of theories," and "No theory is adequate—some are better for some purposes." The authors of the recent study argue that psychotherapy is moving from a more atheoretical eclecticism in the 1970s, which was based primarily on a rejection of psychoanalytic purity, to a more "assimilative integration" in the 2000s, with cognitive therapy as the base of practice, "a firm grounding in one system of psychotherapy, but with a willingness to incorporate/assimilate practices and views from other systems selectively." They contrast this theoretical integrationism with an "evidence-based eclecticism," which would be more empirically oriented. Thus, two varieties of current eclecticism are identifiable: one theoretical (self-viewed as "integrationism") and the other empirical.

Types of Eclecticism

A few different types of eclecticism stand out: the term can be seen as referring to a mixing of theories, or a mixing of methods, or as freedom for individualization of treatment. Another perspective is that it can be seen as open-mindedness to all possibilities *until the data come in,* an empirical eclecticism (consistent with the philosophy of evidence-based medicine [EBM], see also chapter 11). Yet all of these approaches seem unsatisfactory.

The first of these, a mixing of theories, has the problem of determining which theories to choose and how to mix them. Inevitably certain parts of certain theories are left out and others kept, often on unclear grounds. Besides, when there are over one hundred schools of psychotherapy, for instance, the number of possible combinations is endless. Such eclecticism borders on anarchy.

The second, a mixing of methods, might seem more defensible (although eclectic psychotherapists generally deny practicing this kind of eclecticism). The approach would be to ignore theories, focusing rather on the methods used in those approaches and then mixing them as appropriate. Some therapeutic situations might call for empathy (derived from existential theory), others for interpretations (derived from psychoanalytic theory), and others for behavioral interventions. While this technical eclecticism is perhaps more defensible than theoretical integrationism, it again has the problem of specifying when and how such different approaches should be used. No overall eclectic theory so far provides such guidance.

We can also partly justify eclecticism on the grounds of the need for individualization of practice, but only partly. If practice consisted of nothing but individualization, then every single individual would have his own personal diagnosis (or perhaps we would diagnose no one) and his own special treatment. Yet if this were to be the case, we would have to give up on the notion of science, for our practice could not be informed by scientific evidence at all, since such evidence comes only in generalizations about groups of people with similar characteristics (samples). Individualization has to be combined with more general scientific evidence, or perhaps more general theory; individualization pure and simple is idiosyncratic and unscientific. Such eclectics might defend their view, but only on the grounds of giving up any claim to a scientific basis for their work.

Finally, we have empirical eclecticism, perhaps the most common view today.

In this perspective, eclecticism serves as a meta-theory that keeps us open to all possibilities until empirical research provides us data on which to make judgments. This approach can perhaps be appreciated by examining some past and recent discussions in the clinical literature.

Evidence-Based Eclecticism?

One might call the preferred conventional wisdom today an evidence-based eclecticism, the idea being that one should be open to data from wherever they might come. In an early source for this kind of thinking (Yager 1977), eclecticism was viewed as a reaction to psychoanalytic dogmas ("an ideological interest in anything *except* psychoanalytic psychiatry") as well as an atheoretical approach ("an advocacy of eclecticism of treatment procedures resting on no identified single conceptual base"). In this approach, "eclecticism is made necessary not because of how 'reality' is organized [the argument from general systems theory] but rather because of how *we* organize reality; in other words, eclecticism is made necessary by the properties of our own perceptual-cognitive apparatus."[3] Since "the major problem facing the psychiatric clinician . . . human behavior is so complex that any one perspective is insufficient for a full appreciation of all there is to see," the author then goes on to make the key eclectic claim that also underlies the BPS model: "The different perspectives are not necessarily mutually exclusive; in fact, they may complement each other in important ways." He then provides a figure that is an important visual depiction of the assumptions of BPS-like eclecticism (Figure 1).

Figure 1 depicts the different perspectives as similarly valid. There is no particular reason to lean toward one view or the other. In fact, the author states this assumption clearly, arguing that various psychiatric theories can be seen as "approximately of comparable adequacy to explain phenomena. Moreover, none is perfect, and each has its faults and limitations." Writing in the same year as George Engel's first formulation of the BPS, Yager's paper links these views directly to the BPS model: "Given that we can understand complex biopsychosocial phenomena from several perspectives simultaneously . . . and given that at our current level of knowledge no one point of view in psychiatry is totally adequate . . . the psychiatrist's task is to effect the best possible solution for any clinical situation that presents itself, the strategy being decided on only after many possibilities are considered."

How does one settle on the strategy? By thinking about whatever data the psychiatrist possesses and accommodating that information to the patient's preferences and values. Hence, eclecticism is not a specific treatment modality but a method for selecting situationally optimal modalities from among those available

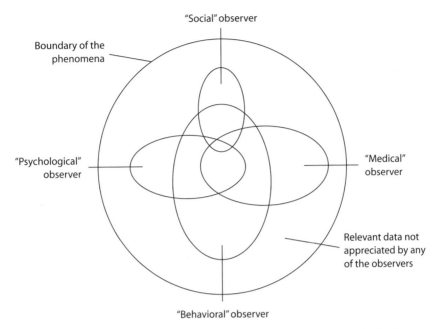

Figure 1. Clinical data processed by four observers with different theoretical orientations (Yager 1977)

in a given case."[4] Yet this author modifies this conceptual eclecticism by saying it is relevant only when clear data are absent: "When the evidence indicates that one mode of treatment is best and that others used concurrently would add nothing or even detract from the value of the most effective treatment, then the best treatment should be used in pure form." It is emphasized that, in psychiatry, our empirical database is limited, hence the frequent need for an eclectic approach, and it is suggested that eclecticism may be most relevant for difficult cases, when single approaches used purely have failed.

Dogmatic Eclecticism

Such eclecticism still coexists uneasily with a wish for an empirically based approach to psychiatry. In response to the paper mentioned above, a young psychiatrist wrote a letter to the editor of the *American Journal of Psychiatry* in which he focused on the notion that in psychiatry each theoretical "framework deserves attention in its own right." The letter writer argued that "human behavior is multi-determined and highly complex, but this does not mean that all of the many expounded viewpoints of human mental illness are correct or that their treatment methods are effective. Just as it is our responsibility as psychiatrists to be eclectically open-minded, we must also be empirically hard nosed. Where possible, we must use viewpoints and therapies that have been demonstrated to be valid." The response to the young critic acknowledged the need for applying scientific data when available, but, "in areas of ambiguity—and it is safe to say that ambiguity remains in much of our field—there is no a priori reason why any frame of reference should command either unquestioning allegiance or out-of-hand rejection." Of course, by using two extreme options, this response did not deal with the real question: Are there ever reasons to give less weight to certain views rather than others on purely *conceptual* grounds? The answer to this question is yes—and it has to be yes; to use an extreme example, would anyone honestly defending "womb therapy" for a patient with schizophrenia? Should it be given a shred of credence, even though there has never been a single empirical study of the topic?

That young letter writer later became a well-known psychiatric geneticist, Kenneth Kendler, who decades later published a conceptual paper taken with great seriousness by the profession (Kendler 2005). Yet, it is perhaps ironic that his recent paper has been widely used to support exactly that BPS eclecticism that he had previously criticized and which he has neither now nor earlier explicitly defended. One might compare another letter to the editor and author response from 2005 to the previous debate of the late 1970s. A recent review of psychotherapies argued for an "informed eclecticism . . . a knowledgeable integration of the several available psychotherapy tools," which was contrasted with "eclectic" psychotherapy, "a potpourri of different activities, fuzzy and unstructured" (Goin 2005). A letter writer challenged any kind of eclecticism: "Research generally shows that adherence to one specific model yields better results than a muddied, mixed [read 'eclectic'] approach. . . . Therapists should equip patients with a kit of finely honed 'tools' for handling symptoms and situations, rather than a hodgepodge of responses. Moreover, no one is really 'knowledgeable' about how best to combine differing treatments. Little evidence is available with which to inform eclecticism. . . . The risk inherent in eclecticism is that therapists will fall into idiosyncratic approaches, as they did in the pre-empirical past" (Markowitz 2005). In reply, the review author cited one authority—Kendler: "Adherence to one particular model may be particularly useful when dealing with psychiatric phenomena that respond to short-term therapy. However, the complexity of personalities and psychiatric illnesses often means that what will prove individually most effective demands integrating in a knowledgeable way an amalgam of methods as currently defined. As Kendler wrote, 'Psychiatric disorders are, by their nature complex multilevel phenomena.

We need to keep our heads clear about their stunning complexity and realize, with humility, that their full understanding will require the rigorous integration of multiple disciplines and perspectives.'" Finished, end of story: *eclecticism ends in dogmatism,* in what Kendler elsewhere criticized as "the great professor principle" (Kendler 1990). ("Professor Freud said" was sufficient in one era, "Professor Krae-pelin said" in another, to imply truth.) Turning to such dogmatic authority to sup-port eclecticism shows, as we saw in the era of Adolf Meyer, how eclecticism often ends in, or is merely a cover for, dogmatism. Further, multifactoriality of mental illness can support eclecticism in the BPS approach, or it may not; it is also com-patible with other non-BPS theories.[5]

The Eclectic School of Medicine

It may be worth noting that eclecticism is not simply a vague epithet: there once was a specific nineteenth-century school of medicine called, proudly, "Eclectic." First a bit of background: Mainstream medicine is called *allopathic,* based on nineteenth-century distinctions. In allopathic medicine, illnesses are treated with opposite in-terventions. (This concept dates back to some Hippocratic maxims [Jouanna 1999].) If patients were hot, they received cold baths. Surgery was obviously an opposite intervention to what was happening naturally (e.g., tumor growth). Homeopathic medicine, in contrast, claimed that "like cures like": symptoms were treated with small doses of drugs that produced similar effects. In the nineteenth century, most doctors fell into one camp or the other; over time, the homeopathic school was displaced by the allopaths in professional medicine. (Some branches of today's "alternative medicine" are essentially a modern continuation of the homeopathic approach.) The eclectic school sought to mediate between the other two: "They consciously borrowed therapeutic principles and practices from both regular med-ical groups and other sectarian ones in an attempt to use all that they thought to be beneficial while rejecting what they considered unsatisfactory" (Connor 1991). The Eclectics originated in 1820s New York, and by the 1890s they had their own Eclec-tic medical schools and hospitals. There were more than 90 Eclectic medical jour-nals by the end of the nineteenth century (the most read of which was titled the *Eclectic Medical Journal*), and they had their own national organization. It is esti-mated that about four thousand physicians were officially called Eclectic around 1900 (compared with about 110,000 allopaths). The treatments used by Eclectics were more similar to homeopaths than allopaths, with much use of botanical com-pounds; unlike homeopaths, though, the Eclectics sometimes used more traditional treatments. For instance, there was a field of Eclectic surgery, whose leader was Andrew Jackson Howe. He was famous for "kitchen surgery," which he performed in people's homes. In 1910, Abraham Flexner's report on "Medical Education in the United States and Canada" sought to implement newer notions of science into medical education, leading to the closing of many allopathic medical schools that had lax scientific standards. The report all but demolished the Eclectic movement, with all Eclectic medical schools closing except one (Cincinnati's Eclectic Medical Institute, which lasted until 1939; Connor 1991).

Eclectic medicine, unlike the homeopathic approach, eventually became incorporated into the more standard allopathic approach. Clearly, the introduction of more strict scientific standards after the Flexner report led to the demise of organized eclecticism. Could it be that eclecticism, in general, reflects absence of science in a field and that, once scientific advances occur, eclecticism disappears?

Pragmatic Eclecticism

Some will still justify eclecticism on pragmatic grounds. Pragmatism as a philosophy has a rich heritage: thinkers such as William James and Charles Sanders Peirce set the standard for American intellectuals. Some authors have argued that pragmatic views support an eclectic approach to psychiatry.

One way pragmatism might support an eclectic view is that pragmatists believe we can only know the truth of things in practice, through using them in our activities. Because our practical activities always involve uncertainties, rather than absolute knowledge, pragmatists then argue that all such knowledge is provisional at best (Brendel 2006). This view derives from Peirce's dictum that "truth is corrected error." Thus, pragmatic eclectic psychiatrists are "fumbling through mistakes to Truth" (Sadler and Hulgus 1992). Yet, this emphasis on the provisional nature of our knowledge, while likely true, is perhaps overdone. If all is provisional, is nothing true? The pragmatic criterion is that "the most important consideration is what form of treatment works" (Simon 1974). Yet as the great British psychologist Hans Eysenck pointed out, such pragmatism needs to be scientifically delimited: we should not be free to choose any approach if we believe that some approaches can be empirically disproven (Eysenck 1952). To paraphrase Freud, truth is not tolerant when it is faced with proven falsehood (Hall and Freud 1960). Such provisional thinking can easily become a justification for indecisiveness, a fatal flaw in practice: this kind of irresolution leaves us in even more eclectic limbo.

The same critique holds for the view that one can integrate differing perspectives with this pragmatic kind of provisional thinking (Sadler and Hulgus 1992). If one holds no views with much certainty, then indeed one might combine different views, but why and how remains unclear. Such mixing of methods, even if labeled "integration," seems little more advanced than the random eclectic mixtures of the past.

Values-Based Eclecticism

Another approach toward eclecticism is to emphasize the role of values, again on pragmatic grounds. In making decisions, as William James famously argued, much of what matters is what we believe; part of making something come to pass is to believe in its coming to pass (James 1956). Pragmatic psychiatrist John Sadler critiques the BPS model as an "anything goes" kind of eclecticism because it pretends to be scientific in a positivistic way, thinking that it simply knows the facts (Sadler and Hulgus 1992). The problem is, as any pragmatist knows, that facts are not simply facts; we do not know data by themselves; we always interpret data through our theories and assumptions. Differences of view, or different ways of understanding a patient or condition, cannot be resolved by appealing to "facts," as empirically minded eclectics would like to do. Integration fails because there is nothing to integrate; the problem is not simply different facts that perhaps can be combined together but also completely different interpretations of the same reality, different "domains of evidence" that cannot be reconciled. Sadler argues then for integration via pragmatic, not positivistic, goals. The issue is "not what is right, but what can I do to help." He thereby emphasizes the importance of paying attention to the patient's values and preferences in the process. This view is, of course, not different from the claim that eclecticism is justified in the need to individualize treatment. While the need for individualization can hardly be gainsaid, the question remains whether we have thereby truly gone beyond "anything goes" practice. After all, if values and preferences vary immensely, would not practice vary immensely? Perhaps there is no problem with this outcome, but then again it would seem there would be little order or rationale to practice beyond trying to meet people's values. And, though the latter is important, it would seem there is a lot more to the science of psychiatry than that perspective. A person might value not taking his lithium, but because he is manic and has ruined his life in the past week by spending until he became bankrupt, his values would not appear to constitute the last word.

General Systems Theory as a Solution

Pragmatism thus seems to fail as a conceptual buttress of eclecticism. To avoid its "anything goes" dissolution, eclecticism must turn elsewhere for theoretical justification, hence the role of general systems theory (GST), which most eclectic theorists, from the 1950s onward, have advocated. Though first developed in 1925 by the biologist Paul Weiss, GST was popularized in the 1930s by Harvard physiologist Walter Cannon (Wynne 2003). In the mid-twentieth century, the prime proponent of this view was Ludwig von Bertalanffy, a German biologist who emigrated to the United States (von Bertalanffy 1974). The key concept of GST, derived as a philosophy of biology, was that the whole is more than the sum of its parts. One cannot explain an organism by simply describing its constituent parts. You cannot understand the gene unless you appreciate other proteins in the cell, or those proteins unless you examine the entire cell, or the cell unless you understand the organ, or the organ unless you appreciate other organs, or all the organs unless you appreciate the behaviors and natural niche of the entire organism. The body is more than the sum of its parts; at its roots, GST is an antireductionist philosophy of biology. These views predated von Bertalanffy, who attempted to put them all together to produce a general philosophy of science, with the view that all special sciences (physics, chemistry, biology, psychology, sociology), just like parts of the body, need to be comprehended within a larger unified view of science. Everything needed to be put together holistically, and this would produce a general scientific theory of all knowledge that would subsume all its disparate components. This was an ambitious task, to say the least, a modern version of the Hegelian wish to achieve Absolute Knowledge. (Much like Hegel, perhaps, one reads pages of GST tracts without appreciating a single concrete idea; yet, despite important insights in both Hegel and GST, such abstruseness should not be confused with profundity).

As a result of the marked interest in GST among psychiatrists, von Bertalanffy was invited to contribute a chapter in the *American Handbook of Psychiatry* (von Bertalanffy 1974). The chapter is thus perhaps the most definitive application of GST to psychiatry in the hands of one of its founders. Unfortunately, von Bertalanffy's essay disappoints. Writing in the midst of the 1960s American counterculture movement, he comes across as a cranky traditionalist, critical especially of behaviorism and humanism. Behaviorism, he argues, tries to reduce humans to conditioned responses; he thought this reductionism was harmful and ignored humanity's cultural uniqueness. Humanistic approaches too had become commercialized, in his view, and oversimplified into nudist EST encounter groups. Von Bertalanffy advocated instead a sober philosophy of biology whereby we accepted that any living organism needs to be understood whole, that we cannot divide a creature into its parts and think thereby that we have understood it, and that this holds even more so for humans because of the human capacity for using symbols.

At times, von Bertalanffy was also critical of psychoanalytic attempts to reduce human psychology to childhood years or basic biological instincts. In sum, he emphasized the importance of the unique symbolic cultural features of humanity and the need for a holistic approach.

In psychiatry, von Bertalanffy viewed the concept of the personality as the hallmark of a holistic approach. While his views can be seen as potentially relevant if seen as arguing for holism in some areas while accepting reductionism in other areas, GST has often been interpreted, or perhaps misinterpreted, as a wholesale rejection of reductionism in all its forms.

Let us turn to see how psychiatric interpreters advocated and applied GST.

Roy Grinker's Eclecticism

Roy Grinker, a key psychiatric founder of the BPS model (see next chapter), viewed GST as the natural biological theory that could explain the multifactorial nature of mental illness: "In my opinion we should approach living human beings as if they existed in a total field of multiple transactions without connotations of significance, hierarchical importance, or conceptual devices called levels. Thereby we avoid the dichotomies of nature vs. nurture, organic vs. functional, lower vs. higher, or reduction vs. extension. Furthermore, we can operationally behave in dealing with multivariable problems as if we really believed in multicausality of both healthy and disordered function" (Grinker 1964b).

Grinker developed a personal relationship with von Bertalanffy, who, in 1971, visited Michael Reese Hospital, headed by Grinker, for one week, and gave the first Roy Grinker Sr. Lectureship there. A few years later, after von Bertalanffy's passing, Grinker gave the first Ludwig von Bertalanffy Memorial Lecture at the annual meeting of the Society for General Systems Research. In this mutual admiration society, it was clear that GST was viewed as the ideal philosophy of psychiatry. Grinker emphasized the importance of a holistic approach to knowledge, recognizing the irreducible nature of complexity and viewing GST as a "meta-theory" that could guide research into specific regions suggested by the overall theory: "This is not to assume that any scientist could cover the entire field, but he could feel comfortable knowing where he was, instead of endlessly riding around in search of boundaries" (Grinker 1976). Grinker emphasized that the attraction of GST was that it provided a theory that allowed psychiatrists, tired of the fights between the two main psychiatric dogmas of biology and psychoanalysis, to give up the search for "the cause" of mental illness and to accept its multicausality.

Grinker was clear that GST itself did not produce data nor was it empirically testable, a critique he courageously made to its main organization: "The Society for General Systems Research and its publication *General Systems* were a mixed bag. Few authors were actually doing research—they philosophized, and many prematurely resolved dilemmas by mathematical equations in a language poorly understood by the empirical investigator" (Grinker 1976). On another occasion, Grinker made a similar point:

> I have tried to show that psychiatric research can be empirical and experimental, controlled, and operational and not dependent on inferences, analogies, or anecdotes. Hypotheses can be derived which are testable. Theory is a different matter. At the present we rely heavily on psychoanalytic theory or on still poorly formulated and defined general systems theory, information theory, or transactional theory. To explain the depth and variety of the interrelationship of soma-topsychosocial facets of the totality of human behavior in process requires a unified theory of human behavior which we have not yet even approached. Integration or synthesis of biological, psychological, and social *theory* is not enough. (Grinker 1964)

Grinker also made the point that GST does not justify the view that we should always and everywhere make holistic connections. It would be a vulgar general systems theory that claimed that reductionism is always bad. Sometimes reductionism is appropriate; other times not. The point of such a theory would be to remind us to look for nonreductionist links between apparently disparate fields; if we find those links, then so much the better, but if we cannot make those links, then the reductionist alternative could be acceptable. This kind of flexibility is often missing in those who view GST as a basis for the BPS model. Such people seem to think that reductionism is wrong, always and everywhere, that everything has to have a tripartite "bio-," "psycho-," and "social" structure, and that the more factors included in a model, the better.

Critiques of General Systems Theory

Others also cast doubt on the power of GST to validate eclecticism in psychiatry. One author writing in the 1970s argued that

> GST falls short of being the sought-after eclectic theory. One shortcoming is that it does not provide a basis for choosing a specific type of intervention. Accord-

ing to GST, intervention at any one level ought to be as good as any other, although we know clinically that this is not true. A theory of eclecticism ought to provide an indication for the level at which to be—and when to switch levels, perhaps—that would be logical and experimentally verifiable. A second problem with GST is that in psychiatry the various levels of possible intervention are less uniform than we might wish. For instance, at the cell-tissue level we deal with concrete and observable phenomena. . . . When we jump to the level of the individual, however, we must add such real but intangible factors as love and hate. The hierarchy looks logical enough on paper, but conceptually there has been a major break at this point. To consider these two levels as open subsystems in interaction with each other is difficult. We have neither the biochemical link nor the psychological link to make them contiguous. (Simon 1974)

These observations are important, perhaps explaining why proponents of the BPS model have been so enamored by the work of research on how conditioned learning leads to neuronal changes in the brain (Kandel 1998).

The author concludes that such an eclectic theory likely will not be found and that eclectic practice must rest on the "art of therapy" (cutely analogized to wine-making; Simon 1974). George Engel, the most famous proponent of the BPS model (see chapter 4), would certainly have disagreed vehemently, because Engel felt that the BPS model made what had been considered an "art" into science. Yet, does the BPS "science" of human psychology and psychiatry, as this critic asked, come close to explaining human experiences like love and hate?

Another critique of the GST was made by a philosopher (also trained in psychiatry) invited to a conference organized by British BPS advocates in 2002 (Malmgren 2005). Perhaps the most objective person in the room, with no previous commitments to the prevailing theory, the philosopher failed to see much value in GST as a basis for the BPS model. As best as one can tell, he argued, GST simply proposes that organisms are best understood as biological systems with a hierarchy of levels of explanation of increasing complexity. These levels interact, but the BPS model does not specify how they interact in medical illness. In their use of GST as a general framework for this model, eclectics provide few specifics on how different levels of understanding an illness directly relate to each other.

GST is broad enough that it in fact says little of specific value to psychiatry except perhaps the general concept of the whole being more than the sum of its parts. Certainly this kind of nonreductionist holism has value, but there is more than one theory of psychiatry that is compatible with it.[6] GST itself can be interpreted dogmatically: everything *has* to be holistic. Yet, sometimes, it would seem, one needs to be reductionistic.

As Grinker admits, because GST is too vague and general for actual research, it is not a scientific theory per se, as philosopher Karl Popper (1959) argued, because it does not lead to testable or refutable hypotheses. Rather, it has a status similar to, at best, evolutionary theory (or at worst, psychoanalysis), what Popper called "a scientific research program" or Grinker's "metatheory"—a philosophy that might provide some general orientation to practitioners but one that does not guide practice or research in any direct way. Perhaps this is why advocates of eclecticism are so drawn to GST: it continues to give them a free hand to do what they like.

Vice or Virtue?

It has been said that eclecticism is a vice in theory but a virtue in practice (Stone 1981), which highlights why so many are attracted to it. But eclectic views cannot survive any careful theoretical or scientific analysis. Deep down, practitioners just want to be free: they believe that their freedom of choice will tailor treatments best to individuals and thus result in best outcomes. Whether or not this is true, it certainly is not scientifically proven, or even likely.

Eclecticism in psychiatry has involved both theoretical and technical eclecticism, as well as the idea of some empirical justification. The GST has been seen as a conceptual model, but it has failed in that role. The various kinds of psychiatric eclecticism, in the end, perhaps share this feature: *As a conceptual theory for psychiatry, eclecticism is a model that views any theory or method as potentially correct, but no theory or method as definitively incorrect.* Hence there is no way to avoid an "anything goes" practice with eclecticism. While seeming open-minded, it is simply an anarchism of mind, and anarchy eventually leads to tyranny, as we will see in the evolution of eclecticism from the psychobiology of Adolf Meyer to the formal biopsychosocial models of Roy Grinker and George Engel.

Riding Madly in All Directions

Roy Grinker's "Struggle for Eclecticism"

Adolf Meyer's psychobiology led to the biopsychosocial (BPS) model that was fully articulated in the 1970s and 1980s by George Engel. But between the two theories, there is a missing link, a part of the tapestry of twentieth-century U.S. psychiatry that historians and psychiatrists have unjustly ignored. In Chicago, at the Michael Reese Hospital, one of Freud's patients was in charge, a man initially trained in neurology who later became a prominent psychiatric researcher. He coined the term *biopsychosocial* and defined and defended the concept throughout the 1950s and 1960s. Unlike Engel (who was an internist), this man influenced psychiatry directly through his role as chair of a psychiatric department and editor of the premier psychiatric journal (the *Archives of General Psychiatry*). The man was Roy Grinker, and one might be justified in claiming that modern psychiatry is more that of Roy Grinker than that of Freud or Kraepelin or Engel.

Roy Grinker the Man

Grinker was a maverick, widely viewed as a curmudgeon, though apparently a lovable one. For thirty-nine years he chaired the psychiatry department at Michael

Reese Hospital, in Chicago (1937–1976), where he trained many psychoanalysts and psychiatrists in Illinois, eighteen department chairmen, and about one hundred professors of psychiatry (including luminaries such as Melvin Sabshin, later medical director of the American Psychiatric Association, to whom *The Diagnostic and Statistical Manual of Mental Disorders,* third edition (*DSM-III;* American Psychiatric Association, 1980), is dedicated; Martin Harrow, a key leader in the field of schizophrenia research who validated Emil Kraepelin's notion of a worsened long-term course in that condition; and Phillip Holzman, the prominent Harvard psychologist who trained generations of researchers in cognitive psychology). One of Grinker's sons, also a psychiatrist, forthrightly describes how Grinker was "both narcissistic and modest," did not believe he was particularly original or creative, and was "intolerant of intellectual sloppiness" (R. Grinker Jr. 1994).

Grinker is perhaps the most prominent psychiatrist who formally and overtly fought for theoretical eclecticism. His advocacy of biopsychosocial eclecticism stemmed primarily from his recognition that psychoanalytic dogmatism was harmful. In this respect, Grinker fought the good fight against dogmatism in an era when few challenged psychoanalytic hegemony. Grinker was one of the few who could have done this, partly because of his own strong psychoanalytic credentials, including his personal analysis with Freud.

Freud's Last Patient?

Grinker's personal experience with Freud is illuminating with respect to its possible impact on Grinker's later eclecticism. It is amusing to read some of the back and forth between Freud and the young Grinker as the unknown American sought to gain access to the master. Though only Freud's part of the correspondence is available in the archives of the Chicago Psychoanalytic Society (Kavka 1999), it appears that Grinker did not shrink from asserting himself, especially in the matter of money.[1] At the time of his death in 1994, Grinker was perhaps Freud's last living ex-patient; he never wrote much about his experience, which his son attributed to Grinker's respect for confidentiality; the other possibility is that Grinker did not get much out of his experience. Perhaps he was unrealistic: only months after their arrival in Vienna, his wife, Mildred, wrote Freud: "A couple of months of analysis have now passed and I see no changes in him" (Kavka 1999). Grinker himself commented that he never felt he discovered anything about himself in a year with Freud (he reported more benefit with later analyses with Franz Alexander and Therese Benedek). He did relate a few anecdotes, about how Freud smoked his cigars vigorously in sessions and puffed smoke all around, about how the dogs would come in and out of the sessions unmolested, about how Freud once tripped and fell, producing a bloody nose, and how Grinker felt too stunned to help the old master (Grinker Sr. 1994). Perhaps what Grinker took away from his experience with Freud was the humanity of the man behind the ideology, the reality of an old Jewish neurologist who boldly proposed creative new ideas and who experimented with new methods. This experience completely contrasted with the buttoned-up high priests of psychoanalysis that would rule the world of psychiatry for fifty years hence. Also, Grinker's own lack of benefit with psychoanalysis in the hands of Freud may have informed his later ambivalence about its therapeutic benefits.

The Struggle for Eclecticism

Grinker saw the road to eclecticism as a struggle, not an easy path of least resistance. This is because Grinker was writing and working in a time when psychoanalytic dogmatism was ascendant and attractive to the best and brightest young minds. To them, the mysteries of psychoanalysis promised to reveal the human psyche completely. Against them, Grinker argued for the limitations of psychoanalysis. The struggle was to open the minds of his contemporaries to different ideas: "We have a hard struggle ahead of us, and I predict that struggle will last for a long time" (Grinker 1964b).

Grinker argued that psychiatry was at an impasse in the shadow of Freud's revolution. The master's metaphors were treated like real entities, and psychoanalysis had suffered from the "monotony of restatement of assumptions. . . . This brave outpost has become a crumbling stockade of proprietary dogmatism" (Grinker 1964b). Freudian orthodoxy had become sterile and rigid; sensing this, psychiatry was "riding madly in all directions," seeking new answers.

In Grinker's day, the struggle against psychoanalytic orthodoxy, and for eclecticism, was initiated and maintained by "social psychiatry," not by the later biological resurgence in psychiatry. By social psychiatry, Grinker referred to the experience of many American psychoanalysts during World War II that one could not ignore interpersonal and real-world social relations in understanding human behavior. Not everything could be reduced to the analyst and his patient, two people, sitting alone in a room, behind closed doors. (A similar critique of psychoanalytic solipsism had been registered by important psychoanalysts, such as Harry Stack Sullivan, Erich Fromm, Erik Erikson, and Karen Horney.) Grinker's social perspective is important, because a generation later, when Engel formally proposed the

BPS model, the impetus to eclecticism would be the resurgence of the biological movement, under the influence of the new psychopharmacology. In both cases, the eclectic thinkers rejected the psychoanalytic orthodoxy that all that mattered was an individual's psychology, taken in isolation from biology or society. Writing in 1964, Grinker was blunt: "psychoanalysis has not become the therapeutic answer." Instead, it was "mired in a theoretical rut vigilantly guarded by the orthodox" (Grinker 1964b).

The Reform of Psychoanalysis

Grinker was uncompromising in his criticism of psychoanalytic dogmatists, head-quartered in the American Psychoanalytic Association (APsA), a view that re-quired a great deal of courage in his day. He noted how the APsA reveled in "its own narcissistic admiration of possessing the sole truth," while critics automati-cally have "transference reactions" (Grinker 1977); how psychoanalysts viewed an-imal experimentation as "degrading" and research as "an intellectual flight from the unconscious," with the result that psychoanalysis "has seriously interfered with clinical research" (Grinker 1966). Psychoanalytic treatment consisted of "gradually increasing fees to lessen . . . minor discomforts," with the concept of "insight" being used in a murky manner: "No one can state clearly what it means, how it is acquired, and how long it lasts" (Grinker 1966). Psychoanalysis, he argued, did not heal the sick at all: "One has to be a fairly normal person to profit from psycho-analysis" (Grinker 1966). Psychoanalysis further harmed attention to observation. "Psychiatric formulations became stereotypes replacing observations and descrip-tions which were depreciated. . . . An unfortunate concomitant of dynamic psychi-atry has been the underemphasis on sound observation" (Grinker 1966).

As psychoanalysis became more and more divorced from reality, would-be pa-tients turned to Indian gurus, transcendental meditation, and other "freaky pseu-doreligions" (Grinker 1977). Yet Grinker was too committed to his first psychother-apist to blame him for the errors of later disciples. Citing another critic, he wrote: "Psychoanalysis by Freud swung the emphasis in psychiatry away from description toward deeper phenomena whose 'meanings were interpreted as causes and whose metaphors were considered as reality' " (Grinker 1964a). "To be a Freudian has come to mean that we accept in a religious sense the words of Freud as scriptures that must be followed directly" (Grinker 1966). Psychoanalysis, turned into dogma, had become both more and less than it might have been: "Its imperfections have not been corrected nor its truths established by testable hypotheses" (Grinker

1977). Grinker emphasized how the early pioneers of psychoanalysis worked by "the seat of their pants," a liberty of method that was killed off by later dogmatism (Grinker Sr. 1994). The future, Grinker felt, belonged to a new eclectic psychoanalysis, rather than a complete dismissal of it.[2]

A New Psychiatric Paradigm?

Grinker interpreted Freud's contribution in the light of Thomas Kuhn's (Kuhn 1996) philosophy of science. Kuhn famously argued that science progresses by revolutionary changes in paradigms, which involved total reconceptualizations, rather than through gradual convincing of the community of investigators of the need for change. The need for a sudden change in paradigm is indicated when scientific work seems stuck, without much progress in the daily work of fact-gathering and interpretation, and when ongoing research tends to conflict with previous theories. At some point, the accumulated conflict blows up the old paradigms. Grinker thought, in 1964, that psychiatry was on the verge of such an explosion:

> In psychiatry our current view of the world of man and his problems is still under the influence of the revolution begun by Freud. . . . Many hitches, however, have been observed in the last decade, and increasing evidences of rigidity are at hand. Stereotypes are rampant, theory is reiterated, and proof is attributed to repetition of hypotheses. But a revolution . . . has not yet occurred. Where and how will this occur? . . . Perhaps it has already begun and is not recognized. All we can say is that some of us know that it is overdue. It may be surmised that, because psychiatry is reaching a state of rigidity. . . . it is now "riding madly in all directions" for solutions—more biology and more sociology, etc. (Grinker 1964a)

Grinker saw the rise of the BPS model as the revolution he had wanted; one can only guess whether he foresaw that, like many revolutions, it might quickly give way to a counterrevolution, a rearguard action to preserve the very psychoanalytic orthodoxy that Grinker had hoped to destroy (see chapter 6).

Grinker's Pragmatism

Grinker's justification for eclecticism is similar to some viewpoints examined in chapter 2: "The number of scientific disciplines involved in psychiatry seems to present a vast array of irreconcilable viewpoints. . . . The problem is how to relate the sciences to each other." He then cites Thomas Mann: "Everything is connected with everything else. . . . We are interested in the whole, or we are interested in nothing." In his discussion of general systems theory (GST), he emphasizes that "one system does not exclude the other, and one alone cannot tell the whole story" (Grinker 1965).

Grinker defined his own concept of the eclectic psychiatrist as follows: He "freely selects from a wide variety of sources what is *available and appropriate*" (italics mine); eclecticism need not mean "disorder, disunity or chaos" as was the case in his day, when psychiatrists rode madly in all directions in seek of some guidance to their confusing field (Grinker 1965). I italicize "available and appropriate" above to highlight that we need to define these terms. If one takes the entirety of his work, it would seem reasonable to argue that he held two criteria as the basis of his eclecticism: pragmatism and empiricism. His pragmatism related to the "availability" criterion; if theories had been developed, then they should be assessed to see if they were practically useful; he even once cited American pragmatist philosopher John Dewey in support of his overall approach to psychiatry. His empiricism related to the "appropriateness" criterion, by which he can be interpreted as meaning that certain theories were tested experimentally and validated. This would be consistent with modern views on evidence-based medicine.

Interestingly, Grinker was not an opponent of specialization, unlike many who propound the BPS model today. He argued that eclectic approaches were especially useful during training in psychiatry but that later specialization was to be encouraged.

The Origin of the Biopsychosocial Concept

Grinker advocated this pragmatic/empiricist eclecticism in a new biopsychosocial view of illness, based on GST. In the rest of this chapter, I examine Grinker's formulation of the BPS model.

First, Grinker upheld a broad definition of psychiatry, beyond simply being a profession that treats severe mental illnesses. "Psychiatry can be broadly defined as a science which deals with the determining factors of human behavior, its variations and vicissitudes, the methods of its analysis, and the means that may be employed to align behavior with optimal personal and social goals." Grinker comments that psychiatry "has expanded above its medical roots to become a science containing a peculiar bio-psycho-social admixture" (Grinker 1965). Grinker applauded this development.

The earliest description of the BPS model as such, in which the label was consciously applied, was a 1952 presentation by Grinker (even earlier premonitions can be found in the work of existential psychiatrist Victor Frankl and psychiatrist John Romano, but Grinker was the first to expound on the idea).[3] Grinker also repeated this presentation of views in numerous articles published in the 1960s, long before Engel's formal articles in 1977 and 1980. Engel too had some earlier allusions to a critique of biomedical reductionism, but I did not find any description of the BPS model, with a use of the term *biopsychosocial,* in Engel's work before the 1970s, whereas such descriptions are clearly available in Grinker's writings from the 1950s and 1960s. In 1952, Grinker put it this way:

> I should like to use another term for the psychiatrist or psychoanalyst differentiating these only in accordance with their special techniques. I should say that they are practitioners in a field of behavior in which they try to understand the psycho-somatic-environmental systems as processes in transaction, within a particular universe or field. The psychiatrist or analyst is usually interpreted most intensely in varying levels of the psychic system. The physiologist or physician penetrates into the depths of activities of the somatic system. The sociologist is more concerned with the interaction of individuals as total persons within various social or environmental settings. It is not possible for any person to fully understand a system from its structural analysis attained by working inside that system alone, however. One can learn more about interrelations between somatic and psychic or between psychic and social systems by making observations *at the boundaries of their intersections* [italics added]. In order to understand more adequately the processes at work in the total psycho-somatic-social field, however, one must understand the processes that go on in transaction among at least three systems by assuming a more distant position outside the system but within the field. (Grinker Sr. 1994)

Only the use of the term *somatic* in place of *bio* would differentiate this description from the later BPS model. Grinker, perhaps more clearly than Engel, emphasized the relevance of knowledge at the boundaries of disciplines and methods rather than from within methods. For Engel, it seemed that the different methods or disciplines or perspectives could be added together to provide the best overall knowledge; this might be called a kind of *additive eclecticism.* Most clinicians seem to unconsciously subscribe to this theory: the more, the better. Grinker was more sophisticated; his view was that the most important knowledge was the kind at-

tained at the intersection of methods; multidisciplinary knowledge was more useful than narrow knowledge within a given field. This might be called *multidisciplinary eclecticism.* (My own view is that they are both wrong; see chapter 16.)

A decade later, Grinker expanded on his early BPS formulation when speaking
to the Association for the Advancement of Psychoanalysis, a group of psychoanalysts who rejected Freudian orthodoxy that he had helped found. In giving the
Karen Horney Lecture in 1966, Grinker wanted to emphasize how useful the BPS
perspective could be for psychoanalysis:

> Those of you who have followed the principal shifts or changes in psychoanaly-
> sis have seen that it began as an open system involving biological motivation,
> conflict and social process. Unfortunately, after the seduction or traumatic the-
> ory which Freud found so congenial in the early days failed, a closed theoretical
> system became the vogue for a long time during which the biological and social
> aspects of human mentation became locked out. . . . Psychoanalysis, except for
> the waning influence of reactionary organizational factions, is now an open sys-
> tem by virtue of the evolution of structural theory, ego psychology, and the con-
> cepts of adaptation. As a result, modern psychoanalysis is a bio-psycho-social
> theoretical structure. . . . The frame of reference of a bio-psycho-social point of
> view has been utilized without sacrificing any of the dynamic concepts which
> psychoanalysis has contributed to psychiatry. (Grinker 1966)

Grinker is thus explicit, despite his frequent criticisms of psychoanalysis, that
the BPS model is meant to *save* psychoanalysis, to allow Freud's theories to survive
in modern psychiatry. Whatever Engel's later goals in medicine, there is no doubt
that in psychiatry, the BPS model came to be viewed in large part, at least by the
1980s, as a savior of psychoanalysis.

Grinker presented his BPS formulation again, in a form more clearly recogniz-
able than its early outline in 1952. Here he also highlighted the roots of the BPS theory in psychosomatic psychiatry, the psychiatric practice that dealt primarily with
medical illnesses with psychological components (see chapter 5):

> The broad term, bio-psycho-social, encompasses all aspects of the living organ-
> ism. It indicates the inseparability of the environment from organic life and the
> relationship between human existence and its social and cultural products. The
> term is not easy to grasp theoretically and difficult to implement operationally.
> With its holistic concepts it is often used to deny the significance of particular
> frames of reference and the importance of one or another variable in health or

illness. I have little use for the pleas to utilize holistic approaches operationally. The scientist has to focus, with a particular frame of reference and from a specified position, on a part of the world of man. Yet unified or holistic concepts in general are important as organizing principles for the understanding of general processes. . . . The same criticism can be applied to the term psychosomatic, which connotes more than a kind of illness. It is indeed a comprehensive approach to the totality of an integrated process of transactions among the somatic, psychic, and cultural systems. . . . In fact, as I stated in 1953, "psychosomatic refers not to physiology or pathophysiology, not to psychology or psychopathology but to a concept of process among all living systems and their social and cultural collaborations. The totality is referred to as the bio-psycho-social system." In 1951, in my presidential address before the American Psychosomatic Society, I stated that "we would fare better if we used the term *behavioral science,* which implies psychosomatic or comprehensive approaches." (Grinker 1966)

Engel never adequately acknowledged Grinker's priority of at least of the term *biopsychosocial,* if not of many of its concepts. One of Engel's close colleagues, writing just after his death, reports that "Engel did not claim to have originated the term 'biopsychosocial model,' so widely associated with his 1977 paper in *Science.* The term was first used, so far as he knew, by an anonymous person attending one of his lectures. Then when he was preparing his 1977 paper, he was told that he needed a memorable label[4] for the concept. He recalled the biopsychosocial term and brought it into the literature" (Wynne 2003). Unless some unknown clinician randomly hit on this term without every seeking acknowledgement, the published psychiatric literature clearly indicates that Grinker had used that term at least twenty-five years before Engel: that "anonymous person" was most likely Roy Grinker.

A Unified Field Theory of Psychiatry

Besides proposing a BPS approach, Grinker tried his hand at developing a general theory of psychiatry, a variation on GST adapted specifically to human behavior. Unlike Engel, he did not claim to have succeeded; instead he admitted that such a unified field theory of medicine (or psychiatry), though profitable, was nowhere to be found in the foreseeable future of our relatively young science:

After World War II, John Spiegel and I, dissatisfied with the overall conceptual approach to psychiatry and unhappy about the available texts, attempted by means of dialogues over a period of three years to develop a generalized theory.

We learned a great deal which we carried with us continually in our separate fields but not enough for the edification of others, so that we abandoned the project. We were convinced, however, that overarching theories had to embrace the entire field from biology to sociology and more.... In 1950 with several kindred spirits we organized a continuous multidisciplinary conference of several distinguished investigators to work "Toward a Unified Theory of Human Behavior." Our first and only report was published in 1956 although we included in this volume only four of our nine conferences. (Grinker 1969)

Unlike Engel, Grinker published proposals for applying the BPS approach to major mental illnesses, such as in a paper on schizophrenia (Grinker 1969).

Grinker thought that no single approach to schizophrenia would prove useful; what was need was a "synthesis of theories." "Theories of psychopathology in general have been zealously defended and considered to be contradictory to each other.... [but] a pure psychogenetic theory is as untenable as a pure genetic theory. There should be complementarity." He then went on to describe "organic" "psychological" and "social" theories of schizophrenia and concluded: "The overlapping and multiplicity of factors places theory of schizophrenia in the currently acknowledged broad biopsychosocial field. Among the terms used to incorporate all the approaches are psychosomatic, multifactorial, field theory, general systems theory, etc. These are much more sophisticated than the usual oversimplified two-system correlations, or the hope-inspiring concept of difficulty in central control, or deficiencies in organizational processes, or the pessimistic statement that schizophrenia is an attempt to adapt to a problem that is insoluble." Grinker then tried to break down the BPS unity into its parts, with a chronological sequence. First, there was the biological diathesis, which led to developmental experiences (including trauma, danger, or dissatisfactions) in early childhood or critical periods of youth, leading to the psychological experience of anxiety. These experiences led to challenges to the biological organism, stresses that reduced the primary symptoms of flat affect, followed by the secondary symptoms of overt delusions and hallucinations. Grinker suggested that the remarkable benefits of medications might be working on the basic biological diathesis to illness. "The process begins ... early ... and is based on primary biological foundations which, even though latent, are probably always part of various transactions during the developmental phases." Grinker argued for the need for complementary, multidisciplinary research "to bring the multiple theories into an understandable and fruitful synthesis," with his suggested chronological integration as one way of trying to put it all together (Grinker 1969).

Another major interest for Grinker was the concept of "normality." Although he admitted that it was difficult if not impossible to define a single positive view of mental health, nonetheless he upheld the importance of studying normality: "I have attempted to interest investigators in the study of healthy or normal persons. I called these mentally healthy male subjects 'homoclites' because of their tendency to conform or follow the common path. How humans get to be healthy should help us understand how and when they deviate into sickness. It is a reasonable postulate that there is no one positive mental health but a variety of healthy, adaptive states" (Grinker 1969). Grinker argued that illness could only happen when enough stress occurs to lead to disease; without stress, there are only variations on normality. Disease occurs from maladaptation to stress. These views are essentially elaborations of similar perspectives derived from Meyer.

The Unknown Grinker

Roy Grinker is the unrecognized founder of the biopsychosocial model and clearly its major advocate within psychiatry. Analyzed by Freud, trained as a neurologist, and a practicing researcher throughout his life, Grinker was one of those rare persons who eclectically combined in himself the disparate parts of psychiatric practice. Perhaps this unique background is also what enabled him to be uniquely aware of the limits of such eclecticism. This humility appealed to a profession hungry for eclectic permission to be free of dogma. It remained for George Engel to take up the banner of a formally presented model of illness, which would become the new theoretical core of the mental health professions to the present.

CHAPTER FOUR

A New Model of Medicine

George Engel's Biopsychosocial Model

A theory is a reflection of the person who created it. George Engel, the person generally acknowledged as the founder of the biopsychosocial (BPS) model, once described how he, his twin brother, and his older brother, Lewis, were strongly influenced by their uncle, Emanual Libman (1872–1946), a prominent New York physician (whose visitors and patients included Einstein, among others). "All three of us soon enough found ourselves preoccupied with figuring out just what it was he did and why he was so famous and sought after" (G. L. Engel 1992). Lewis became a scientist, not a doctor, later chair of biochemistry at Harvard. Engel notes that he and his twin brother, Frank, were more impressed by their uncle's clinical reputation and reported skills than by his scientific reports. They both became doctors. Engel wondered whether the clinical aspects of medicine (as opposed to the more technical scientific parts), in which his uncle demonstrated such skill, could likewise be conducted scientifically. In 1941, when doing a research project with psychiatrist John Romano, Engel concluded that it was possible to take a scientific approach to the medical interview that might elucidate the human aspects of medicine. "From that time on my whole outlook, professional and scientific, was never again to be the same. The human dimensions of medicine had for me at last become accessible to scientific inquiry, just as had the heavens by the invention of the telescope. One could be scientific at the bedside after all!" (G. L. Engel 1992).

This was at the source of Engel's efforts with the BPS model: Engel wanted to make a science of the clinical bedside experience between doctor and patient. Whether he succeeded or not is at question.

Engel the Internist

Engel, whose theory is at the heart of modern psychiatry, was not a psychiatrist and never trained in psychiatry. He trained and practiced in internal medicine, with a special interest in gastrointestinal diseases. His first publications were about nerve metabolism, and his main interests had nothing to do with major mental illnesses.[1] Indeed, in his early career, he was a self-proclaimed biological reductionist: "He dismissed most of what psychoanalytic psychiatrists had to say as 'laughable' and as 'hogwash' " (Brown 2003). Even though he later became sympathetic to psychiatry and psychoanalysis, he never developed a strong interest in mental illnesses per se. In fact, "his main diagnosis of interest" was ulcerative colitis.[2] Other areas of research were psychogenic pain and the effect of psychological states on gastric secretion in babies with gastric fistula. He wrote a book on fainting and two popular texts on "Psychological Development in Health and Disease," and "The Clinical Approach to the Patient," but nothing specifically on psychiatric conditions. (Of about 175 original articles and reviews, Engel never once wrote about mania or schizophrenia.) He attended the Johns Hopkins University medical school in the 1930s, an era in which the iconic influence of William Osler was vivid. Like Osler, Engel's most important early medical activity involved autopsies, arranged by his uncle with a prominent forensic pathologist (one summer Engel observed more than three hundred autopsies; Ader and Schmale 1980). Whereas Osler used this experience to popularize the "clinicopathological" method in medicine and to introduce an organ-based, disease-oriented science to medicine, Engel went in the other direction, emphasizing, with his BPS model, the importance of the clinical interaction above laboratory tests or pathological examination.

Engel the Psychoanalyst

In the 1940s, Engel met psychiatrist John Romano in the course of his training; he would follow Romano throughout his career, first when Romano became chairman of psychiatry at the University of Cincinnati and later at the University of

Rochester (where Engel spent the bulk of his life). Encouraged by Romano, Engel took an interest in the psychological aspects of gastrointestinal illness and, consequently, engaged in formal psychoanalytic training for five years in the 1950s in the Institute for Psychoanalysis in Chicago (which, run by Franz Alexander, was the center of psychosomatic medicine).

Thus, Engel, the man, was an internist who sought to better understanding gastrointestinal illness through the use of psychoanalytic ideas. Some of his clinical views are clearly outdated due to their psychoanalytic orthodoxy: For instance, in 1956, he theorized that headaches in persons with ulcerative colitis were due to "strong conscious or unconscious aggressive or sadistic impulses." "Bleeding," in ulcerative colitis, he argued, "characteristically occurs in the setting of a real, threatened, or fantasized loss, leading to psychic helplessness" (Shorter 2005). Engel would later move away from such simplistic psychoanalytic ideology, but he never completely left behind the psychoanalytic influences that were a key aspect of his intellectual formation.

In fact, he made it clear that he wanted to forge "a liaison between internal medicine and psychoanalysis." A close colleague who knew him up to his death noted that "Engel long remained dedicated to psychoanalytic theory" writing a highly critical review in 1971, for instance, of John Bowlby's work due to "faulty understanding of psychoanalytic theory" (Wynne 2003).

Engel the Psychosomatic Specialist

In his clinical work at the University of Rochester, Engel mainly focused on what is now called consultation-liaison (CL) psychiatry, that is, assisting medical colleagues in treatment of nonpsychiatric patients. Hence Engel's work was primarily directed toward understanding the psychological aspects of medical conditions, rather than the biological aspects of psychiatric conditions. Engel's influence is perhaps deepest in the CL subspecialty in psychiatry, as witnessed by recent issues in his honor in the prominent CL journal *Psychosomatics and Psychotherapy* (Fava 2000).

Engel is often lionized by his followers, especially in Rochester (Frankel, Quill, and McDaniel 2003), as a revolutionary who bucked the tide. In fact, he was simply following the psychiatric crowd. Until the 1970s, he was anything but unpopular. His text, *The Clinical Approach to the Patient,* published in 1969 was widely read and received rave reviews in the *Annals of Internal Medicine.* He had many fellows and students in his CL program. He traveled all over for invited lectures at the most prestigious universities. In these addresses, he tended to emphasize the importance of psychological stress and particularly psychoanalytic notions in illness; in this work, he was following the psychoanalytic crowd.

Historians have noted that his influence paradoxically began to wane as he became more famous (Brown 2003). The 1971 edition of *Cecil's Textbook of Medicine* (Beeson and McDermott 1971), for instance, cites his work and ideas on ulcerative colitis in detail; by the 1979 edition, he was hardly cited, and psychosomatic notions were largely dismissed. Engel was disturbed by these changes; to some extent, his classic 1977 paper on biopsychosocial concept, where he first clearly formulated the model, was a *cri de coeur* and a declaration of war, aimed at a field that was putting him aside. He was complaining about medicine becoming more biological, but his impact was strongest in psychiatry, where his psychoanalytic friends saw the BPS model as a defense against biological psychiatry.

It should be emphasized that Engel was bothered not just by medicine becoming more biological but specifically by the decreased attention to *psychoanalytic* ideas. For instance, current proponents of the BPS approach often point to the field of psychoneuroimmunology as an example of the model in action in research; yet Engel was disturbed by this new field. He opposed the advance of "animal models, stress studies, and psychoendocrine bench research" as they displaced "earlier, psychoanalytically grounded clinical studies" (Brown 2003). Despite the claims of his current disciples, Engel was committed to a psychoanalytic orientation, and not just the generic value of psychology, in understanding illness.

The popular mainstream psychosomatic researcher and teacher of the 1950s to 1970s era became, at the end of his career, the theoretician of the BPS model. Despite immediate acclaim for his 1977 paper and his growing influence in psychiatry, Engel, increasingly disillusioned in his final decades, felt clinical medicine was only paying "lip service" to the BPS model (Brown 2003). Still, Engel was never an outsider or rebel: by the 1990s, the majority of medical schools had incorporated the BPS concept into their educational programs (Brown 2003). Despite such mainstream acceptance in education, however, the BPS model has not been enacted easily in practice or research. Engel tended to blame the powers that be; he never blamed the model itself.

Birth of the Formal Biopsychosocial Model

The first explication of Engel's views related to the BPS model dates to 1951, when he gave a lecture, perhaps not surprisingly, to Roy Grinker's department at the Michael Reese Hospital in Chicago. While this date precedes the first description by Grinker of the BPS approach in writing in 1952, Engel's paper was not published until 1954 in a book edited by Grinker and in revised form in 1960 in a medical journal (titled "A Unified Concept of Health and Disease"; G. L. Engel 1960).[3] Many attribute the true origins of the BPS model in Engel's work to this paper from the 1950s; however, it is far less clear and overt in its views than Grinker's work from that era, and, as a matter of historical record, Engel never uses the phrase "biopsychosocial" or refers to it as a model or directly contrasts it with biomedical models, whereas Grinker used the phrase first in writing clearly in 1952 and repeatedly thereafter into the 1960s, as demonstrated in the previous chapter. Clearly, Roy Grinker is the father of the BPS model, though Engel popularized and extended it to the medical profession as a whole.

The 1977 Science Article

Engel wrote two classic papers in which he laid out his mature view of the BPS model. The first, published in *Science* (G. L. Engel 1977), was directed to a general medical audience; the second, published in the *American Journal of Psychiatry* (G. L. Engel 1980), was directed to psychiatrists.

In the *Science* article, Engel first provided the psychiatric context for his views, especially the rise of a biological tendency in psychiatry in the 1970s:

> At a recent conference on psychiatric education, many psychiatrists seemed to be saying to medicine, "Please take us back and we will never again deviate from the 'medical model.'" For as one critical psychiatrist put it, "Psychiatry has become a hodgepodge of unscientific opinions. . . ." In contrast, the rest of medicine appears neat and tidy. . . . But I do not accept such a premise. Rather, I contend that all medicine is in crisis, and, further, that medicine's crisis derives from the same basic fault as psychiatry's, namely, adherence to a model of disease no longer adequate for the scientific tasks and social responsibilities of either medicine or psychiatry. . . . Psychiatry's crisis revolves around the question of whether the categories of human distress with which it is concerned are properly considered "disease" as currently conceptualized. . . . Medicine's crisis stems from the logical inference that because "disease" is defined in terms of somatic parameters, physicians need not be concerned with psychosocial issues. (G. L. Engel, 1977, p. 129)

Biological psychiatrists have a simplified notion of disease, he continues:

> The dominant model of disease today is biomedical, with molecular biology its basic scientific discipline. It assumes disease to be fully accounted for by devia-

tions from the norm of measurable biological (somatic) variables. It leaves no room within its framework for the social, psychological, and behavioral dimensions of illness. The biomedical model not only requires that disease be dealt with as an entity independent of social behavior, it also demands that behavioral aberrations be explained on the basis of disordered somatic (biochemical or neurophysiological) processes. Thus the biomedical model embraces both reductionism, the philosophical view that complex phenomena are ultimately derived from a single primary principle, and mind-body dualism, the doctrine that separates the mental from the somatic. (G. L. Engel, 1977, p. 130)

Instead, Engel concluded, we should consider psychological and social factors as key to all illness:

The boundaries between health and disease, between well and sick, are far from clear and never will be clear, for they are diffused by cultural, social, and psychological considerations. The traditional biomedical view, that biological indices are the ultimate criteria defining disease, leads to the present paradox that some people with positive laboratory findings are told that they are in need of treatment when in fact they are feeling well, while others feeling sick are assured that they are well, that is, have no "disease" . . . By evaluating all the factors contributing to both illness and patienthood, rather than giving primacy to biological factors alone, a biopsychosocial model would make it possible to explain why some individuals experience as "illness" conditions which others regard merely as "problems of living" . . . It is the doctor's, not the patient's, responsibility to establish the nature of the problem and to decide whether or not it is best handled in a medical framework. (G. L. Engel, 1977, pp. 132–33)

He next examined grief, which can be viewed as both a problem of living, to be handled by psychotherapists outside of a biological medical framework, or as a disease, treated within a medical framework. It is up to the biopsychosocially aware physician to make these distinctions: "The psychobiological unity of man requires that the physician accept the responsibility to evaluate whatever problems the patient presents and recommend a course of action, including referral to other helping professions. Hence the physician's basic professional knowledge and skills must span the social, psychological, and biological . . . Is the patient suffering normal grief or melancholia? . . . The patient soliciting the aid of a physician must have confidence that the M.D. degree has indeed rendered the physician competent to make such differentiations" (G. L. Engel, 1977, p. 133).

He concluded by noting that medicine had become "cold and impersonal" and that increased interest in primary care medicine grew out of unhappiness with "an approach to disease that neglects the patient." He argued that psychiatry was making a mistake in moving away from its psychological orientation. He cited Freud and Adolf Meyer and general systems theory as intellectual sources for his view: "One of the more lasting contributions of both Freud and Meyer has been to provide frames of reference whereby psychological processes could be included in a concept of disease" (G. L. Engel, 1977, p. 196).

Engel's *Science* article thus lays out all the basic elements of the BPS model. His critique of the narrow biomedical model appears to have had the most influence in general medicine. A recent paper in a family practice journal summarized Engel's critique of biomedicine as follows:

1. A biochemical alteration does not translate directly into illness . . .
2. The presence of a biological derangement does not shed light on the meaning of the symptoms to the patient . . .
3. Psychosocial variables are more important determinants of susceptibility, severity, and course of illness than had been previously appreciated . . .
4. Adopting a sick role is not necessarily associated with the presence of biological derangement.
5. The success of the most biological of treatments is influenced by psychosocial factors, for example, the so-called placebo effect.
6. The patient-clinician relationship influences medical outcomes . . .
7. Unlike inanimate subjects of scientific scrutiny, patients are profoundly influenced by the way they are studied, and the scientists engaged in the study are influenced by the subjects. (Borrell-Carrio, Suchman, and Epstein 2004)

The importance of treating the person not just the patient, the importance of psychosocial factors in illness, the importance of the physician-patient relationship—these are of course those aspects of the BPS that Engel presented to the larger medical audience. He also upheld, as we have seen, more directly psychoanalytic perspectives on the nature of the psychological factors related to medical illness, as well as the nature of the relationship between doctors and patients.

The 1980 *American Journal of Psychiatry* Article

Now let's turn to how Engel formulated his model more specifically for psychiatry (G. L. Engel 1980), derived from an invited lecture to the 1979 annual meeting of the American Psychiatric Association in Chicago.

In this article in the *American Journal of Psychiatry* (*AJP*), Engel first restates the problems of the biomedical model, which was (and in general medicine still is) the predominant conceptual model against which Engel proposed the biopsychosocial concept as an alternative. In the biomedical model, the "crippling flaw" was that "it does not include the patient and his attributes as a person, a human being" (G. L. Engel 1980). Engel was not making simply a humanistic claim here. He was claiming that the BPS was a better "scientific model" than the biomedical model and that it was a better model not only for practice but also for education and medical research.

Engel begins at the meeting of doctor and patient. "The most obvious fact of medicine is that it is a human discipline, one involving role- and task-defined activities" of doctor and patient. The patient is in "distress," with a concern about illness; the doctor is competent to assess that possibility and to engage the patient in cooperating in treatment if needed. Thus "in the everyday work of the physician the prime object of study is a person," and the medical process involves "an ongoing human relationship" with "behavioral and psychological forms, namely, how the patient behaves and what he reports about himself and his life." The biomedical model reduces all psychological and social aspects to "physico-chemical terms" due to its "mind-body dualism." "Hence the very essence of medical practice perforce remains 'art' and beyond the reach of science." Engel argues that the BPS model is more *scientific* than the biomedical model, because it can scientifically take into account psychosocial components that the latter ignores.

Engel emphasizes that a model for medicine needs to focus on "what the physician does" not "what the bench scientist does." He argues that biomedical reductionism errs in having as its gold standard the experimental paradigm in which the bench scientist controls all aspects of the environment except one, which he can then test experimentally. Obviously, this is impossible in any human medical encounter. (Although one could claim that large replicated randomized clinical trials approach this experimental ideal; Engel never apparently discussed this issue.)

Engel goes on to explain the nature of systems theory as a nonreductionistic approach to biology (see chapter 3): "Nature is ordered as a hierarchically arranged continuum, with its more complex, larger units superordinate to the less complex, smaller units. . . . Each level in the hierarchy represents an organic dynamic whole. . . . Each system implies qualities and relationships distinctive for that level of organization, and each requires criteria for study and explanation unique for that level. In no way can the methods and rules appropriate for the study and understanding of the cell be applied to the study of the person as person or the family as family."

Engel then gets into the core of his paper, which is the application of the model to a patient case. It is fascinating that he chose someone with myocardial infarction as his case-a medical, rather than a psychiatric, diagnosis. One might view this as a strength: if the BPS model could work in a medical case, it must be even more applicable to psychiatric cases. Presumably this is how the paper was appreciated by readers of the *AJP* in 1980. One could also view this as a weakness: the central conceptual model of psychiatry is based on an article in which the key example is a patient with a heart attack, not depression or psychosis.

Engel's case, Mr. Glover, is a 55-year-old married man who has a second heart attack at work. He initially ignores the symptoms, denies having them, and is ultimately persuaded by his employer to go to the emergency room. There appropriate cardiac care interventions are made, and he improves. After an inexperienced resident fails to obtain an arterial blood puncture after repeated attempts, the patient gets more concerned and anxious, and then has a cardiac arrest, followed by defibrillation and recovery. Engel contrasts two approaches to the case: In the biomedical reductionist approach, the problem is the myocardial infarction. The patient's feelings and reactions are not relevant and are largely ignored. The person *is* the disease. In this approach, the fact that he demonstrated an attitude of denial to his symptoms and fear about his fate is irrelevant, as is his reaction to the failed arterial blood punctures that contributed (presumably) to his subsequent cardiac arrest. In contrast, the BPS approach would take into account the importance of these psychological factors from the outset and, thus, might have prevented the second cardiac arrest by also attending to his psychological reactions. According to Engel, the BPS approach would see the person as primary and view the heart muscle ischemia within the hierarchy of systems ranging from the cells to the muscles to the nervous system to the person to the doctor-person relationship to the community and society. The biopsychosocial physician would have this whole in view, as opposed to reducing the illness to the muscle level.

Engel published nine figures in his article, which are all variations on this systems hierarchy, seven of them demonstrating the effects of events or interventions at different system levels in this case. Clearly, he was trying to make a point.

The key to the case seems simple: The biomedical physicians did not attend to the patient's psychological feelings and reactions; the biopsychosocial physicians would have. Yet how is this different from simply being humanistic and treating patients as persons, as Osler instructed? Engel later claims that this BPS approach is not simply the application of humanism to medicine. At least in this case, the practical difference for the patient's care seems minimal.

Only in the ninth figure do we get a sense of where the BPS model might go beyond humanistic medicine in practice. There, at the top of his hierarchy, Engel
places the "society-nation" and writes that a result of Mr. Glover's case, there might
be "social policies re[garding] toll of heart disease and rehabilitation." Engel is arguing that the BPS model would provide a rationale for going beyond the care of
an individual patient to thinking about social and public health approaches to illness. In this respect, the model can provide a rationale for public health concepts,
in which illness is prevented or attended to at the level of social factors that predis-
pose to illness, as opposed to simply being treated at the individual level of the sick
patient. Except for that minor change to the ninth figure compared to the preceding eight, Engel does not expand on this connection of the biopsychosocial approach to a public health model in medicine. Instead he mainly emphasizes the
psychological aspects of an individual's reactions to illness and the social aspects
of his relationships to his medical team. These aspects of the case are less convinc-
ingly unique or improved by adhering to the BPS model, compared with simple
medical humanism (see chapter 12).

The Attack on the Humanities

Engel appears to anticipate such a reaction by emphasizing that the BPS model is
scientific. He argues against the antithesis set up between science and the humanities, which he sees as based on an overly reductionist view of science: "For the
biopsychosocially oriented physician this is not merely a matter of compassion and
humanity, as some would have us believe, but one of rigorous application of the
principles and practices of science, a human science" (p. 543). He approvingly cites
a paper by Margaret Mead on "human science." The application of humanistic approaches to medicine would be too subjective and individualistic for him: "For the
biomedically trained physician, judgments and decisions bearing on interpersonal
and social aspects of patients' lives commonly are made with a minimum of information about the people, relationships, and circumstances involved and with even
less knowledge and understanding of basic principles underlying interpersonal
and social transactions. By and large the physician reaches decisions on the basis
of tradition, custom, prescribed rules, compassion, intuition, 'common sense,' and
sometimes highly personal self-reference. Such processes . . . remain outside the
realm of science and critical inquiry. Not so for the biopsychosocially oriented physician" (pp. 542–43).

I spell out in chapter 12 how Engel's *antihumanism* is a key, and often unknown, feature of his BPS model. Here it is relevant that Engel never spells out in what way the BPS physician is more scientific about the psychological and social aspects of illness than the humanistic physician. In the case of psychiatry, readers of *AJP* would know the implication. Many, one can imagine, concluded that psychoanalytic views were more scientific than common sense or intuition, and thus the BPS was a justification for the utility of those psychoanalytic notions. Certainly Engel's personal history would suggest that he would have been sympathetic to that interpretation. It is interesting, though, that nowhere in his *AJP* article, in contrast to his *Science* article, does he mention Freud or psychoanalysis or indeed Meyer or any other intellectual antecedent to his views in psychiatry. Given that he touched on that issue in the *Science* article, which was intended for a general scientific audience, it is curious that he ignored it in his primary paper for a psychiatric audience.

Whatever Happened to the Biopsychosocial Physician?

Engel addresses one last issue that would later loom large in the decline of the BPS model in psychiatry-the problem of expertise:

> Some argue that the biopsychosocial model imposes an impossible demand on the physician. This misses the point. The model does not add anything to what is not already involved in patient care. Rather, it provides a conceptual framework and a way of thinking that enables the physician to act rationally in areas now excluded from a rational approach. Further, it motivates the physician to become more informed and skillful in the psychosocial areas, disciplines now seen as alien and remote even by those who intuitively recognize their importance. And finally, the model serves to counteract the often wasteful reductionist pursuit of what often prove to be trivial rather than crucial determinants of illness. The biopsychosocial physician is expected to have a working knowledge of the principles, language, and basic facts of each relevant discipline; he is not expected to be an expert in all. (Engel 1980, p. 543)

Here Engel gets to what would prove to be a key problem in the later application of the BPS model to psychiatry (see chapter 10). The fact is that many clinicians have seen this approach as a reason to mix differing methods but to never be very competent, not to mention expert, in any one of them. This is especially the case when the BPS model has been used as a rationale for a single physician treater as opposed to split treatment with multiple mental health professionals.

It is also striking that Engel claims that the BPS approach "does not add anything to what is not already involved in patient care." This formulation brings out most clearly how the approach was interpreted, in psychiatry especially, as a defense of the 1970s status quo-specifically, a defense for the continued importance of psychotherapies (in particular, psychoanalysis). Incorporating the BPS model into psychiatry was seen as a conservative move, a counterreaction to the psychopharmacology revolution.

Another way of noting how the BPS model has been part of the psychiatric status quo for the past three decades is to examine textbooks from the 1970s. For instance, in the prime text of that era, the 1974 second edition of the *American Handbook of Psychiatry* (Arieti 1974), the first volume is entitled *The Foundations of Psychiatry*. It includes an invited article on the relevance of general systems theory to psychiatry by Ludwig von Bertalanffy and numerous articles on psychological aspects of mental illness ("The Personality," "The Concept of Psychological Maturity," "The Life Cycle," "The Family," "Infant Development," etc.). In a section on "The Various Schools of Psychiatry," of nine schools described, five are psychoanalytic ("Classical," "Adlerian and Jungian," "British Psychoanalytic," "American Neo-Freudian," "Miscellaneous Psychoanalytic"), three involve other psychotherapy approaches ("Psychobiological," "Existential," "Behavior Therapy"), and one is hard to categorize ("Organismic") but seems to represent a Gestalt-oriented approach. No school is described for the traditional medical-biological-objective descriptive approach that dates back to Kraepelin and Griesinger and their contemporaries. There is not, and never has been, much "bio" in the BPS in psychiatry.

The Return of the Repressed

At the end of Engel's paper, after his references, empty space in the *AJP* is filled with a "Notice to Clinical Investigators" that reads thus: "Under program support from the Foundations' Fund for Research in Psychiatry, three research laboratories have been designated as resource groups for clinical investigators doing blood level research with antianxiety, antidepressant, and antipsychotic drugs. Investigators who seek to establish the reliability of their methods or those who wish to participate in a proficiency testing protocol should contact the appropriate group listed below."

Perhaps no better coda could be provided to the political relevance of Engel's article. The BPS model was being proposed at just the time that a biological upswing was taking place in psychiatry. This was no coincidence.[4]

What Was Original about Engel?

There was no really innovative component to Engel's thinking; the catchiness of the term *biopsychosocial model* (which the historian Edward Shorter [2005] suggests may be the relevant point) was originated by Grinker, as was the idea to link the biopsychosocial model to the philosophical idea of general systems theory. The rejection of mind-brain dualism had also been central to the ideas of previous psychosomatic eclectics (see the next chapter).

What was unique about Engel was that he took this holistic, eclectic, psychosomatic notion of mankind that had sprung up in a corner of psychiatry and used it as a weapon to fight what he viewed as the dogmatic biological reductionism of modern medicine. Engel brought the BPS model to all of medicine, as opposed to focusing on psychiatry.

Time would show that Engel's main impact was back in the psychiatric world from which he had originally derived his ideas.

CHAPTER FIVE

Before and After

Precursors and Followers of the Biopsychosocial Model

The rise of the biopsychosocial (BPS) model, as exemplified by the careers and works of Roy Grinker Sr. and George Engel, cannot be understood separately from the rise of the perspective of psychosomatic psychiatry (psychiatry related to medical illness), which grew out of Freud's work. While Freud applied his theory to hysteria and other psychological syndromes, it was perhaps logical that others would apply it to medical syndromes. Among the first to do so in the United States was neurologist Smith Ely Jelliffe.

Smith Ely Jelliffe and Psychosomatic Disease

At the turn of the twentieth century, Smith Ely Jelliffe wrote perhaps the first paper to specifically argue for a psychological cause for a medical illness (psoriasis; Burnham 1983). Many of Freud's early supporters were neurologists rather than psychiatrists. For decades, Jelliffe was coeditor of the *Journal of Nervous and Mental Disease*, the most prominent neurological journal in the United States, with psychiatrist (and long-time head of St. Elizabeths Hospital in Washington, D.C.) William Alanson White. In the 1920s, though, Jelliffe's journal lost its place of honor to the new *Archives of Neurology,* partly due to the rift between those who supported an organic approach to neurology versus Jelliffe's psychosomatic tendencies. Like Freud, Jelliffe was a private practitioner, seeing many patients in his busy Manhattan practice, whom he treated with a mixture of traditional neurology and psychoanalytically informed psychotherapy (in fact, he wrote one of the first technical handbooks about the methods of psychotherapy). Jelliffe had been introduced to Freud and Jung's ideas at the same time, when the two were still allies, and after Jung's schism, Jelliffe was always seen by Freudians as vacillating between the two. Ultimately, it is most likely Jelliffe was a true eclectic, unable to fully accept or reject any one Freudian group. He found expression for his eclecticism in the idea of psychosomatic illness, in which Freud's notions could be mixed even with physical disease. Freud himself was cool to the idea, though he did not actively oppose psychosomatic views. Freud's closest personal disciple who went in the same direction was Franz Alexander (a mentor to both Roy Grinker and George Engel), who moved to Chicago and formally established psychosomatic training.

Franz Alexander's Psychosomatic School

Like Jelliffe, Alexander argued that psychoanalytic constructs were the cause of some physical illnesses. This view led to great opposition from many internists and neurologists. Grinker provides a good example:

> It was at the University of Chicago where Dr. Alexander was placed in the unfortunate position of giving a seminar concerned with the relationship of psychoanalysis and medicine to members of the Department of Medicine and various invited, but essentially hostile, guests. On one particular day Alexander recounted a case history illustrating the dynamics of constipation. At that time, and perhaps even yet, he contended that constipation was based on a syllogism, "inasmuch as I do not receive, therefore, I do not have to give." He told the story of a young lady who had developed constipation shortly after her marriage to a man who paid little attention to her. In his management of this case Alexander spoke to the husband and pointed out that her constipation was a reaction to his lack of attention. Whereupon the guilty husband immediately became solicitous, purchased a few red roses and gave them to his wife. Immediately after she received the first gift since their marriage her constipation miraculously disappeared. This was too much for the Department of Medicine and marked the beginning of Alexander's end at the University of Chicago! (Grinker Sr. 1994).

Those early forays were seen as too simplistic. Grinker, Engel, and others revised Alexander's approach to emphasize that psychological factors were important, though not solely causative, in physical illness; they contributed to physical illness, along with other important biological factors or mechanisms. Grinker directly analogizes the term *psychosomatic* to the term *biopsychosocial*, thus clearly showing how the BPS model grew out of the psychosomatic wing of psychiatry. Just as Grinker argued that the term biopsychosocial was holistic and did not imply the reduction of any aspect of life to another, so too the term psychosomatic did not imply a reduction of somatic illness to psychological cause, as Alexander had implied: "It is indeed a comprehensive approach to the totality of an integrated process of transactions among the somatic, psychic, and cultural systems . . . as I stated in 1953, 'psychosomatic refers not to physiology or pathophysiology, not to psychology or psychopathology but to a concept of process among all living systems and their social and cultural collaborations. The totality is referred to as the bio-psycho-social system' " (Grinker 1966).

Thus, the main source of the BPS model is psychosomatic medicine, concerned with medical illnesses with psychological components. It has been little discussed whether a model derived from this small corner of the psychiatric profession is appropriate for the entire broad range of mental illnesses.

Multicausality of Illness

Consistent with the origins of biopsychosocial concepts in psychosomatic psychiatry, the BPS model has continued to have its most dedicated defenders in the camps of consultation-liaison psychiatry and psychosomatic medicine. Giovanni Fava, for instance, defines Engel's BPS model as based on a "multifactorial view of illness" as follows:

> It allows illness to be viewed as a result of interacting mechanisms at the cellular, tissue, organismic, interpersonal, and environmental levels. Accordingly, the study of every disease must include the individual, his body, and his surrounding environment as essential components of the total system. The various social factors involved may range from the socioeconomic status (e.g., poverty, nutritional deprivation, loss of social support) to toxic environmental exposure, in a truly ecological perspective. Psychosocial factors may operate to facilitate, sustain, or modify the course of disease, even though their relative weight may vary from illness to illness, from one individual to another, and even between 2 diff-

erent episodes of the same illness in the same individual. Susceptibility to disease may be influenced by activation of a variety of central nervous system pathways. (Fava and Sonino 2005)

He adds that the "doctrine of multicausality" is the "core postulate of current psychosomatic medicine" and the latter is "by definition, multidisciplinary." Fava describes clinical applications of this approach as

the integration of psychological interventions . . . and psychopharmacology. . . . It appears to be particularly warranted in the following clinical situations:

1. Refractoriness to lifestyle modifications guided by primary care or other non-psychiatric physicians.
2. Presence of psychological disturbances (e.g., demoralization and irritable mood) or of psychiatric illness (such as major depression or panic disorder)
3. Presence of abnormal illness behavior interfering with treatment or leading to repeated health care utilization, such as illness denial or hypochondriasis.
4. Impaired quality of life and functioning not justified by the medical condition (Fava and Sonino 2005).

If we focus on the second point above, the claim is that most psychiatric illness can be understood with the BPS model and require both psychotherapy and psychopharmacology.

Elsewhere, Fava (1992) defines psychosomatic medicine as concerned with

1. The assessment of psychosocial factors affecting individual vulnerability, course, and outcome of any type of disease.
2. The holistic consideration of patient care in clinical practice.
3. The specialist interventions to integrate psychotherapies in the prevention, treatment, and rehabilitation of medical diseases.

Clearly, the psychosomatic approach to medicine and psychiatry is based on a holism and antireductionism that is also at the core of biopsychosocial eclecticism.

The Case of Monica

Engel's writing supports the view that psychosomatic concepts are central to the BPS model. He noted that "there are those who hold that all diseases are psychosomatic, those who hold that only some are, and those who hold that none are"

(G. L. Engel 1967). And then he expressed some skepticism: "Strictly speaking, there can be no 'psychosomatic diseases,' just as there can be no 'biochemical diseases' or 'physiological diseases.' Rather diseases have their psychosomatic and biochemical and physiological components or aspects. And if we agree on a broad definition of disease as referring to failures of the organism to adjust for longer or shorter periods of time to changes in the environment, internal and/or external, then the psychosomatic approach is concerned with the ways in which psychological and somatic factors interact in the whole sequence of events that constitute a particular disease experience" (G. L. Engel 1967).[1] He then described a classic case from his research:

> [In the case of] Monica, the 1½ year old infant with a gastric fistula, we demonstrated that gastric hydrochloric acid secretion correlated with the intensity of interaction with the experimenter. When Monica was relating actively, either with pleasure or rage, gastric secretion rose, as it did when she was reunited with the experimenter. On the other hand, when she disengaged, including falling asleep, acid secretion fell, most strikingly so in the profound withdrawal reaction to a stranger. Now these findings appear to be in keeping with the classical psychoanalytic concept of orality, that is that external object relating is modeled on the first nursing and feeding experiences, external objects being dealt with as if they are literally to be ingested. On the strength of these data and this theory we predicted that with psychic development beyond the oral stage, behaviour and gastric secretion would become dissociated as psychic activity becomes more autonomous. This prediction has been born out in a comparable study of Doris, a 4½ year old, also with a gastric fistula. . . . In contrast to Monica, Doris' gastric secretion correlated not with the intensity of the relationship, but with the effort to secure or hold the relationship. Now in spite of the temptation by some to relate such findings to the pathogenesis of peptic ulcer, I would contend that no such inference is justified. . . . [But] the suggestion of a relationship between gastric acid secretion and the vicissitudes of object relating is of fundamental importance for the theory that object relating constitutes *one* category of psychological processes operating at the psychosomatic interface. (G. L. Engel 1967)

Engel goes on to note that while we can associate psychological and somatic processes in time as occurring simultaneously, causality is hard to establish. "In my opinion there is still not available a scientific system whereby relationships across the psychosomatic interface can be established. . . . We have some good physiological measures, and we have some psychological categories and theories; but it remains unclear how to connect the two groupings. . . . Certainly we have little idea at the present how to relate phenomena across frames of references. It is in this sphere that we need a theoretician of the caliber of Darwin or Einstein. My belief is that a completely new system remains to be evolved" (G. L. Engel 1967). Engel's biopsychosocial model fails as such a system, as does von Bertalanffy's general systems theory: both simply pointed out the relevance and importance of such interactions across levels, but exactly how such interactions happen was left completely unresolved by both theories. (Grinker, in contrast, admitted his failure to invent such a grand unified theory.) One might view the work of Nobel laureate Eric Kandel on the physiology of learning in *Aplysia* as a first step to demonstrating such interactions in reality (Kandel 1998), but that work is still a far cry from what need. We still await our Darwin and Einstein; perhaps we should give up the wait.

A Conference on the Biopsychosocial Model

So much for psychosomatic medicine before BPS founders Grinker and Engel. Now, after the passing of these two men in 1992 and 1994, respectively, we live in an era of their disciples. How do they promote or understand the BPS model?

One gets a sense of the contemporary state of the BPS approach in general medicine from a 2005 conference in London, sponsored by a nonprofit organization devoted to spreading that doctrine (White 2005).[2] The conference attendees were mostly members of the choir, already believers in the BPS approach, which gave the proceedings a somewhat uncritical air. Nonetheless, some critical comments were also voiced, especially in the audience discussion period.

The conference began with its chair pointing out the dualism of medical practice, in his case using the Institute of Psychiatry in London as an example (Wessely 2005). It is located next to Maudsley Hospital, a psychiatric hospital, and across the street sits King's College Hospital, a general hospital. The chair noted that few clinicians work on both sides of the streets.[3] The worlds of mental and physical illness are by and large separated. The head of the nonprofit group emphasized how the BPS model was an extension of, not a replacement for, the biomedical model and that the discussion at the conference would focus on chronic medical diseases, for which the BPS model might be most relevant. The subtext throughout the conference was to ask two questions: (1) is the BPS model valid (which most attendees assumed to be the case) and (2) if it is valid, why has it not gained more influence in general medicine?

A Philosopher's Doubts

Of about a dozen lectures, only one was given by a philosopher (also trained in psychiatry), who was also among a minority of persons there not professionally committed to the BPS model (Malmgren 2005). He noted that proponents of the BPS model unanimously rejected mind-brain dualism, but that dualism is not so easily set aside: philosophical attempts to reduce mind to brain have been fraught with problems; nonreductionist alternatives generally recognize mental states as separate from brain states and distinguish among first-, second-, and third-person perspectives. In many ways, the philosophical concept of "supervenience" is equivalent to the philosophy of disease based on the general systems theory that Engel and Grinker upheld. But a note of caution is in order: if one factor (say a mental state) is supervenient on (emerges from but is not reducible to) another factor (say a brain state), then one cannot speak of the joint effects of the two. In other words, saying that Nassir and the physical body currently sitting at the computer are writing this book is meaningless, because the person "Nassir" is supervenient on the physical body that is sitting at the computer at this moment. Similarly, if we say that schizophrenia may be the result of abnormal dopamine pathways and a certain personality predisposition, and it turns out with future research that the personality predisposition is manifested in those abnormal dopamine pathways, then we are simply saying the same thing twice.[4]

I have not read this warning anywhere else in the BPS literature: the notion that the BPS model is relevant because mental illnesses are *so* complex may in fact be a mirage. We may be making things more complex than they are, by counting factors over and over again that in fact are supervenient expressions of one factor. Horror of reductionism lies at the root of the BPS approach. It could be that, by refusing to reduce complexity, we thereby create complexity.

The discussion that followed was enlightening, with the attendees apparently taken aback by the philosopher's critique of the assumptions of the BPS model and perhaps unfamiliar with the philosophical terminology used. The chairman expressed the unease: "My impression was that all you thought of Engel's work is that this is simply another version of common sense intuition and that it lacked any methodological rigour or clarity. Is that right?" The philosopher's response:

> I didn't use common sense in a pejorative way. George Edward Moore at Cambridge raised common sense to the standard of philosophy. If something is a commonsense opinion and you can't come up with any good counterarguments,

then it is probably true. And I haven't found any powerful arguments against the biopsychosocial model in its crude formulation that mental and social events influence and interact with biological events. But Engel's ideas are not philosophically very deep. Specifically, he does not explain how such an interaction can take place, taking into account the laws of physics and chemistry. What was new in his approach compared with the common sense perspective is the systems theory approach, which does not solve the just-mentioned problem. (Malmgren 2005)

The point here is that even if one does accept the BPS approach to mental illness as philosophically correct, it is superficial: it tells us little of value. There are important truths, and there are superficial truths. The BPS model may be a superficial truth: the claim that all illnesses have biological, psychological, and social components, if true, is a trivial truth—it does not explain the more important question of exactly how they interact to produce illness and corollary questions of how to assess the relative importance of different components regarding etiology, pathogenesis, and management (see chapter 7).

Despite this clear warning that the BPS model is a philosophical lightweight and a reiteration of the mistake of seeing two factors as "interacting" when in fact they might be one and the same factor seen from two different perspectives, this critique seemed to go over the heads of the participants. The chairman summarized thus: "I don't know if it possible to sum up what we have discussed so far, but I'll try. We began by seeing Engel in his appropriate historical perspective, from within the problems in psychiatry and the crisis of confidence in medicine. Yet it remains a source of some contention within psychiatry. . . . We have also heard the philosophical rationale for mind-body interactions and that there are no serious philosophical objections to the BPS model, if properly updated" (White 2005, p. 36). No objections, one might suppose, if one prefers not to hear them.

The Benefits of Reductionism

Other presentations at the conference made the important contemporary link between the BPS model and public health. A key one was provided by Michael Marmot (2005), a prominent epidemiologist who has shown that social factors appear to be independent causative factors for chronic medical illnesses such as coronary artery disease. The thrust of his paper was to show that empirical research has demonstrated the relevance of purely social causes to some medical illnesses. Yet in the discussion, he was criticized for seeing social causes as always working through biological mechanisms, instead of looking for two-way interactions. Marmot's response is an example how, even in the hands of its sympathizers, the BPS model is not helpful in research: "I take your point completely," he replied, "but as a scientist who looks at relationships between variables A and B, I do need to constrain my thinking. Otherwise I cannot move: I am just paralysed by complexity." *Paralysis by complexity*: this might be a good summary of how the BPS mind-set is impeding contemporary psychiatric thinking.

Epidemiologist George Davey Smith (2005) made matters worse when he pointed out the benefits of reductionism: "contrary to the view that embracing complexity always gets us closer to the truth, much of what we know about disease actually suggests that the utilization of rather simple models of linear causality is often appropriate, particularly when we are considering ways of improving population health." Even though Engel grudgingly admitted that biomedical reductionism had led to progress in the past, his attacks on it led his disciples to interpret the BPS model as implying that complexity is the case—everywhere and always. Smith was reminding us that this is not true. He made the point that the perspective of complexity tends to be more prominent when we have *less*, not more, understanding of a disease. His key example was peptic ulcer, a classic psychosomatic illness that even Engel had used as an example of the multicausal nature of disease. It now appears that perhaps the key etiological factor is *Helicobacter pylori* infection. Davey Smith noted how he once gave another colleague a paper about peptic ulcer and how it was heavily influenced by psychological stress and asked the colleague if the paper was a fair description of what people think; the colleague responded that but for some stilted language, such was the case, and then Davey Smith revealed that the paper dated to 1850 and was written about general paralysis of the insane (GPI, or neurosyphilis); Smith had simply inserted "peptic ulcer" everywhere for GPI. In other words, BPS-like explanations of illness, the idea of "mental stress" somehow interacting with personality, have always been common rationalizations for conditions that later turn out to have straightforward biological causes. Indeed this apparently reasonable eclectic approach to explaining illness can hinder, rather than help, medical knowledge. Davey Smith noted that though *H. pylori* was introduced as a cause of peptic ulcer in 1983, the first hypothesis of bacterial associations was put forward in 1875, some researchers advocated antibiotic treatment for peptic ulcers as early as 1948, and an antibiotic received a patent for such treatment in 1961. The infectious disease approach, which would later prove effective, was ignored for about a hundred years, partly because physicians were wedded, following Engel's views among others, to a BPS model that deemphasized biological factors (Davey Smith 2005).

After casting doubt on the validity of the BPS model as an explanation of the etiology of diseases, Davey Smith also expressed wry skepticism about its humanistic utility: "When writing about a myocardial infarction patient whom he had seen, Engel stated, 'In the end, whether the patient lives or dies, the BPS model further provides the physician with the conceptual tools to clearly think and plan the implications of the cardiac arrest.' If I have a heart attack [states Davey Smith] I want to be treated by a doctor who cares about whether the patient lives or dies. I'm not really concerned about whether the doctor has the above-mentioned conceptual tools" (Davey Smith 2005). Engel had earlier responded to this criticism, with some impatience, as merely reflecting the harmful reductionism of the biomedical model. Davey Smith's point is more profound: he makes this claim only after showing that the BPS model was wrong, and harmful, in the peptic ulcer story. His claim is this: It is not enough to claim utility of the BPS model in the interests of humanistic medicine; it has to mean more. Engel claimed it provided a more valid assessment of the nature of illness. This is not the case even in conditions that have been seen as traditional psychosomatic conditions, like peptic ulcer. Why, then, give up a biomedical model appropriately seasoned by medical humanism (as with Osler) for the BPS model (see chapter 12)?

Biology versus Psychology

George Davey Smith's paper generated the most extensive and engaged discussion of the conference. The chairman began by noting: "That was a powerful and uncomfortable paper. . . . [but] there is a popular and seductive Whiggish view of medical history in which we move implicitly from unknown diseases which are thought to be psychiatric and as we become brighter, better scientists they are finally accepted into the pantheon of real diseases. You should remember that there is an opposite trend as well. . . . You ignored the history of visceral proptosis, floating kidney, autointoxication, or focal sepsis, for example. There are also lots of other things that are seen as very clearly organic and which switch the other way" (p. 99). Marmot agreed: "It is easy to look back and say, 'Gosh how silly they were in the past to think all these silly thoughts; aren't we clever now!' . . . Your logic seems to be to seize on the notion of stress and say that people were silly about it before, therefore we should never think about stress ever again. . . . Research has advanced beyond the examples you cite" (p. 100). Davey Smith responded that, while he thought that psychosocial factors were relevant to the etiology of many illnesses, especially psychiatric, they were not yet shown to be "direct causes" but rather influences on "the distribution of known exposures." He argued that "susceptibility has been overplayed and exposure has been under-appreciated in social epidemiology" (p. 99). In other words, Engel and Grinker always emphasize the multicausality of mental illness; yet Davey Smith is suggesting that this should not be interpreted as multiple direct causes of illness: for instance, severe major depression is not the result of biological abnormality X in the brain + psychological cause Y + social cause Z. Rather, social factor Z perhaps increases exposure to biological cause J. One can intervene either at the level of social factor Z or biological cause J, depending on which aspect is more amenable to intervention, but to ignore the ultimate biological cause may be counterproductive. Again the history of peptic ulcer disease and *H. pylori* may be instructive; perhaps social factor Z sometimes increases exposure to *H. pylori;* even so, *H. pylori* is still key to the causation of the illness and a major point for intervention, while social factor Z is secondary and only contributory to the extent that it affects exposure to *H. pylori.*

A final comment from the audience concluded that Davey Smith had raised the need to distinguish different aspects of the BPS model, such as etiology versus treatment: "We may have to differentiate in the BPS model between aetiology, where it is a weaker kind of model, and intervention for complex diseases such as back pain, cardiac syndromes, and depression" (p. 101).

Seen as a "devil's advocate" (p. 226) at the overwhelmingly probiopsychosocial meeting, perhaps Davey Smith could take solace in the fact that the devil was, after all, a fallen angel who had glimpsed the truth.

Disease versus Illness

Another response to Davey Smith was provided in the meeting by one of the few attendees who had worked with Engel. This author focused on the distinction between disease and illness:

The disease is the externally verifiable evidence of a pathological state and the illness is the patient's perception of ill health. We have to come to terms with the limitations of psychosocial factors in explaining the aetiology of clearly established chronic disease, such as heart disease or arthritis. Once we have done this, we can focus more on adaptation and management using psychosocial parameters. . . . [In the case of peptic ulcer] I see some of my patients treated against *Helicobacter pylori* and they come back complaining of ulcer pain. My guess is that they are *H. pylori* negative and endoscopically have no ulcer, because they have successfully been treated. Yet the pain persists: "illness without disease." The fact is that ulcers and pain do not always correlate. Instead, a patient may have functional dyspepsia. . . . The challenge is to recognize what we mean by illness and disease. When we look at the biomedical model, there is no question that there are biological determinants that explain disease. The assumption is, however, that the disease explains the illness in a linear way, which then explains the outcome. We accept that there could be environmental exposures that will modify this and there might even be psychological overlay that can affect the outcome. But the point is that it is a linear model, where the disease explains the illness. What about illness without disease? . . . From a healthcare systems model, physicians are confronted with illness, not disease, particularly in primary care. This is what we have to understand, study, and treat. That is not to say we do not study and treat disease, but we do not want to blur the boundaries. (Drossman 2005)

This author, though repeating some of Engel's views, cedes some territory Engel was not willing to cede. Though Engel did distinguish between illness and disease and saw the BPS model as related to the patient's experience of illness, he also saw it as relevant to the etiology of disease. Certainly, many of the psychiatric advocates of the BPS model see it this way: they view the three BPS factors as etiologies of mental illnesses. If we accept that etiology of disease is mainly biological and that the BPS model is most relevant in terms of the individual's subjective experience of illness, we are making a separate claim that neither Engel nor Grinker made (and we are not far from Osler's view of medicine; see chapter 12).

The Rochester Tradition

Another source, an edited volume written by Engel's colleagues and students from the University of Rochester (Frankel, Quill, and McDaniel 2003), will help us understand how the BPS model is now used by his disciples in the United States.

In a section on clinical practice (Epstein et al. 2003), for instance, the authors identify "six central aspects of the biopsychosocial approach": "Eliciting the patient's story and life circumstances; integrating the biological, psychological, and social domains; recognizing the centrality of relationships in providing care; understanding the physician; focusing the model for clinical practice; providing multidimensional treatment." Looking at these six factors, which seem reasonable, two questions come to mind: first, which of these six are unique to the BPS model versus other models? And second, what do they mean? It appears to me that four are not unique to BPS, at least compared with a humanistic biomedical model: The BPS model is not the only approach to medicine that cares about the individual's story and life circumstances; subjective experience is important in the Oslerian tradition as well (chapter 12); as for psychiatry, many other approaches attach much import to the subjective experiences, especially Karl Jaspers's empathy-oriented phenomenology (chapter 17), as well as Freud's free association method (Havens 2005).

We are left with two unique claims about the BPS approach: that it integrates the three domains and provides multidimensional treatment. Regarding integration, the authors basically emphasize that the clinician needs not only to diagnose disease but also to pay attention to the individual's subjective meaning of illness and to examine "the fabric of the patient's life" in their relationships. They then provide a case of a 32-year-old chain-smoking prison guard who has chest pain, extensively worked up by non-BPS physicians as possible variants of cardiac illness, while a BPS approach soon determined that they represent panic disorder, responding to antidepressant treatment. In other words, the authors try to explain the integration of the three domains by emphasizing the need to pick up psychiatric conditions with somatic presentations. Except to restate the old psychosomatic perspective—that some psychiatric conditions have physical symptoms—it is not clear how this explains, in a general sense, the integration of biological, psychological, and social factors as a model of health and illness.

Turning to the unique second BPS factor of multidimensional treatment, the authors present two cases: one of a 58-year-old man with HIV on a complex medication regimen, who had chronic pain requiring narcotics, lived with and cared for his elderly mother, and had some cardiac risk factors that led to complicated decision-making regarding his medications. The second case was of a 9-year-old boy with sore throat but a mostly negative physical examination, whose mother asked about penicillin and was educated about the lack of need for such medications. The authors emphasize that in these cases, the physician needs to understand the individual's feelings about medications and tolerance of uncertainty and the physician's own feelings about using narcotics for pain or antibiotics for nonspecific infectious symptoms; the "human connection" was key to providing care in these cases. It remains unclear to me how this description of multidimensional treatment goes beyond the other aspects described above of paying attention to relationships in treatment, including the person's subjective experience. Nothing unique to the BPS model is described here that is not also found in other approaches (chapter 12).

The authors also highlight what they see as misconceptions of the BPS model (Epstein et al. 2003): First, believing in a biopsychosocial approach does not mean that there necessarily are psychological or psychoanalytic causes for medical illness but rather that there are multiple factors, including the psychosocial. This perspective has come to be widely associated with the BPS model; only in its early psychosomatic origins did it have the psychoanalytic causative flavor. Second, "the biopsychosocial approach is not prescriptive. There is no single clinical method or treatment approach advocated." This is an important point, since sometimes the BPS model seems to be misinterpreted as privileging the psychosocial domains, or even one specific perspective, particularly psychoanalytic theory. Other misconceptions cited are the idea that the BPS approach is similar to alternative medicine (reminiscent of Engel's wish to be seen as advancing science rather than humanism or simply holistic approaches), that its utility is limited to primary care as opposed to other specialties, and that it is costly in time and money. The authors do not so much refute these criticisms as object to them.

The Postmodernist Turn: On Psychiatric Bullshit

Biopsychosocial eclecticism agrees with another turn of mind: postmodernism. Postmodernism is not as complex a notion as might appear to some readers: one might initially be intimidated by all those French names (Foucault, Derrida, Lacan) and those long and numerous books. Perhaps the key notion behind postmodernism is most simply expressed by Harry Frankfurt's recent philosophical critique of it, titled *On Bullshit* (Frankfurt 2005). Frankfurt did not use that term merely to heap abuse on postmodernism; he expresses, with notable philosophical seriousness, that postmodernism is all about bullshit, i.e., the belief that all ideas are junk, merely means of persuasion, efforts to ideologize power; all this because there is no truth. We need have no special respect for words and ideas because they do not signify truth; words and ideas become bullshit.

I do not mean to be pejorative; I am merely reporting the language that Frankfurt, a senior Princeton philosopher, has used, a perspective widely shared by many sober philosophers, not to mention his many readers.

Postmodernism, then, is the notion that the "modernist" goal of discovering the truth through reason and science ("the Enlightenment project") has failed; our claims to truth and knowledge, whether through science or democracy or other ideologies, are merely culturally relative opinions, with economic and political sources. Our ideas (to adapt Marx) are a mere superstructure to our culture.

This way of thinking has taken root throughout Western culture. It began with the Romantic movement of the nineteenth century, a protest against the rise of science, culminating most explicitly in the work of Nietzsche at the turn of the twentieth century. Many commentators think that it became associated with a certain nihilism, especially after the shock of the Great War of 1914–1918, which seemed to put the lie to the modernist notion of endless peace and prosperity. It seemed even more vindicated by the rise of Nazism in the heart of the most modernist, scientific, rationalist Western nation—and the horror of the Holocaust that seemed to be the result of technology applied to evil purposes (Bloom 1988).

Nietzsche's nihilism began to take root in interwar France, especially with the influence of Alexandre Kojeve (1980), who mixed this postmodernism with Marxism; it took off in postwar France, spawning a generation of thinkers who fully formulated the postmodernist ideology, perhaps foremost among them Michel Foucault (1988). The student revolts of 1968 are often seen as the practical flowering of the postmodernist rejection of liberal democracy and all its rationalist-scientific ideologies. The neoconservative reaction of the 1970s and 1980s followed, and the last few decades have been the setting of "culture wars" between postmodernism and conservatism among Western intellectuals.

This background sets the stage for another cause and consequence of the BPS model. By the 1980s, Western societies were ready for a way of thinking that gave up pretenses to truth, one that allowed for so much flexibility that almost anything could be true. Postmodern sensibilities had become comfortable with this approach, and the BPS model fit it perfectly.

The connection was not explicit until recently, however. As Ralph Waldo Emerson said, philosophies can become part of our bones. We do not need to read thinkers to learn the ideas; when those ideas are part of the climate of cultural opinion, we imbibe them with our mothers' milk. Commentators on Kojeve (Drury 1994) have noted that one consequence of postmodernism could be eclecticism. If there is no truth, and the world cannot be fundamentally altered in any "right" way, then any approach can make sense.

Engel and Pragmatism

This intuition, now deeply embedded in American culture (Bloom 1988), explains the continuing attraction to the BPS model for many psychiatrists today. This link is best seen in a special issue on this approach in the journal *Philosophy, Psychiatry, and Psychology*. There, one author attempts to link Engel's work to the philosophy of pragmatism (Lewis 2007). As discussed in chapter 2, this attempt fails. Pragmatism as a philosophy should not be confused with the meaning of the English word. *Pragmatism* in English implies simply being practical and abjuring theories;

pragmatism as a philosophy involves the perspective that the truth is known by its results. This is the basic concept, at least as initially proposed by Charles Sanders Peirce, but also as the philosophy was later developed by William James and John Dewey. The basic notion is that the truth is not some abstract external entity to which our ideas correspond; rather the truth is known by its results in the world of experience. Peirce analogized this view to the work of scientific experiment: we don't speculate about theories; we test them and see their results in an experiment. Peirce believed that there are truths and that our scientific experiments get us closer and closer to those truths.

The pragmatic author above (Lewis 2007) takes a different view (more in line with James and Dewey) that there is no independent truth; our pragmatic theories are thus only about what is useful, not what is true. Hence the direct link to Engel: there is no truth, therefore we can use any aspect of the biopsychosocial perspective that we wish to emphasize. As described previously, this is just "anything goes" eclecticism again, the kind of anarchy that leads to tyranny, the return of dogmatism under the cloak of eclecticism. The author of this paper appropriately noted the limitations of Engel's view, such as his hostility to humanism and literature, but did not note how committed Engel was to the psychoanalytic paradigm. The recognition of Engel's limits turns into an even more nebulous expansion of the BPS model, a boundaryless postmodern eclecticism, well expressed when the author argues that adding pragmatic philosophy to Engel will enhance the BPS model and make it even more comprehensive:

> Because "mind" is the level of meaning systems, phenomenology, narrative, and psychoanalysis become obvious tools for understanding at this level. In addition, Dewey's metaphysics take the phenomenological and narrative critiques of Engel one step further. Dewey's plateau of "mind" goes beyond "consciousness" to also include cultural influence on the individual identifications and experiences. As such, this level opens beyond phenomenology, narrative, and psychoanalysis to include cultural, social, and literary studies of political and cultural identification. These rich interdisciplinary domains open further on to the critical interpretive tools of feminist studies, race studies, postcolonial studies, disability studies, queer studies, religious studies, and other area studies. (Lewis 2007, p. 307)

Where is it going to end? I have respect for some of the work in all of these postmodernist fields; I just do not think that psychiatry will be much improved by adding them to Engel's limited BPS perspective. The work of Cornel West, for instance, is specifically identified in this paper as being relevant to a pragmatic reinterpretation of Engel (Lewis 2007). I respect West's work and admire him as a person, but I do not think his philosophy will provide the major conceptual turn we need in psychiatry. If we needed proof that the BPS model has no boundaries and that it can be taken anywhere and everywhere, we need only glance at this article.

An Attempt to Rehabilitate Meyer

In the same special issue, another author (Double 2007), an explicit proponent of applying postmodernism to psychiatry (Double 2002), tried to defend the BPS model by returning to Adolf Meyer, seeking to rehabilitate his thinking. This writer performed a service in showing how Meyer was an extremely obsessive peacemonger, a person just unable to disagree with anyone. For instance, in the Meyer Archives at the Johns Hopkins University, letters exist in which Meyer struggles with a critique of the behaviorism of John Watson; he writes multiple drafts, each less critical than the other, until his final letter is hardly critical at all. Toward the end of his life, he expressed his regrets in a note that he apparently wrote for himself: "Why did I fail to be explicit? . . . I should have made myself clear and in outspoken opposition, instead of a mild semblance of harmony. . . . What was it that failed to get across? Did I pussyfoot too much?" (Double 2007, p. 334).

While noting this weakness, the author argues that Meyer's theory was coherent and correct and that he only failed in being explicit enough about it. We should return to the BPS model more explicitly, the paper concludes, and all will be well. In response to my published critique (Ghaemi 2007), the author argues that one cannot critique Meyer's work as eclecticism, as I do, because it was intellectually coherent: "he did not combine together different sources to create an unintegrated philosophical and conceptual understanding. His theoretical position was internally consistent" (Double 2007). I agree that he had a coherent and internally consistent theory: the theory of psychiatric eclecticism in its "psychobiology" formulation. I am not claiming that eclecticism is incoherent at all times (though sometimes it is); I claim that when not incoherent, it is simply wrong. Adding and mixing methods does not get one inherently closer to the truth. If one accepts the postmodernist position, as this author does, there is no truth, and psychiatry becomes all about what is useful, not what it true, devolving into "negotiation" with patients, as Meyer explicitly proposed.

From Postmodernism to Politics

One of the insights of postmodernism (anticipated by Marxism) is that politics affects science. The postmodernists err by concluding that science is *nothing but* power politics and that claims to scientific truth are no more valid than other opinions. Because it is true, however, that science has a political context, we should supplement the conceptual discussion of the BPS model with an analysis of its political impact on the battle between the two dogmas of psychiatry.

CHAPTER SIX

Cease-fire

Ending the Psychiatric Civil War

In Beirut during the 1970s, Christians and Muslims tore their nation apart in a bloody civil war. There was a boundary that could not be crossed, except at the risk of one's life-the Green Line; on one side lived Christians, on the other Muslims. For more than a decade, violence ruled.

A Psychiatric Civil War

The world of 1970s psychiatry was not dissimilar, with physical violence replaced by verbal conflict. On one side of the grand divide stood the psychoanalysts, the Old Guard, with their own informal politburo of leaders; on the other stood the Young Turks, the biological renegades, an "invisible college," scheming and plotting to take over the profession. What was at stake was not only our understanding of mental illness but, to put it frankly, power (Foucault was partly right here). For decades, one could not be a chairman (women were rarely chairs) of a department of psychiatry without being a psychoanalyst. Patronage of academic jobs, control over training the younger generation, access to university resources and government funds-all these were in the hands of the psychoanalytic profession. In the biological laboratories of the National Institute of Mental Health of the 1950s, some government-salaried psychiatrists began to challenge psychoanalytic dogmas and dared to study the brain in relation to mental illness. This group, headed by Seymour Kety, thereafter expanded its reach when Kety and a group of his disciples obtained jobs on the Harvard faculty and at Massachusetts General Hospital (MGH). The way was paved for them because Stanley Cobb, the former chair at MGH, while supportive of the psychoanalytic approach, also believed in the importance of biological methods. Kety's arrival in Boston coincided with a gradual disaffection of younger residents with traditional psychoanalytic teaching, as observed at that time in the premier psychiatric residency in the nation, the Massachusetts Mental Health Center ("Mass Mental"). Mass Mental had been headed for decades by Elvin Semrad, a charismatic teacher who had imbued hundreds of residents with his skepticism for diagnosis, biology, and pharmacology and with an overriding belief in the importance of the human doctor-patient relationship (augmented with psychoanalytic concepts). It is ironic that the leaders of the biological Young Turks came mostly from Semrad's later Mass Mental students (most prominently Gerald Klerman) or across town at MGH from Kety's new students (most prominently Eli Robins).[1]

At first, the major centers of psychiatric training and practice (like Washington, New York, Los Angeles, and Chicago) remained firmly in psychoanalytic hands. (To this day, those large cities have notable cadres of practicing psychoanalysts, unlike most other small or medium-sized American cities). Like Mao's communist revolution in 1940s China, the biological rebels would have to start in the countryside and gradually surround the cities. Perhaps the most important node in the rebellion was St. Louis, where Eli Robins went after his training at MGH to become psychiatry chairman at Washington University. He linked up with a like thinker, Samuel Guze, and trained a cadre of biologically oriented leaders that would remain prominent for decades to come. The Washington University school also produced the first new empirical research on diagnostic criteria, returning to Emil Kraepelin's basic notions augmented by genetic, course, and treatment studies. Robins and Guze published a classic paper, "The Reliability and Validity of Diagnostic Criteria for Schizophrenia" (Robins and Guze 1970), that might be compared, if readers will forgive the continuing analogies, with a Communist Manifesto for the biological revolution. It remains to this day the core of our conception of psychiatric nosology, of what make a diagnosis valid. In that paper, Robins and Guze argued that because no single gold standard exists to validate clinical diagnoses in psychiatry (brain pathology cannot provide the "right" answers for clinicians), we must validate psychiatric diagnoses using multiple independent lines of evidence. They defined these four categories as symptoms (phenomenology), genetics (family history), course of illness (age of onset, number of episodes, etc.), and treatment response (or laboratory tests if available). (This is a somewhat altered version of their original paper, updated to its current usage.) With these tools, they went about demonstrating that definitions of mental illnesses could be established and tested.

This diagnostic research proceeded below the radar screen of mainstream psychiatry, as psychoanalysts went about their business in the 1960s and 1970s, more or less oblivious to the brewing rebellion occurring in the U.S. heartland. What was happening in St. Louis seemed an anomaly; New York and Chicago remained firmly focused on the vicissitudes of the Oedipus complex.

The Rise of Psychopharmacology

A second force would later combine with this diagnostic revolt to tear down the structure of psychoanalytic psychiatry. In 1949, an isolated provincial Australian psychiatrist discovered lithium. First John Cade took lithium himself to make sure it was safe. Noticing no effects, he gave it to manic, depressed, and schizophrenic individuals and noted that it completely and specifically cured mania! Here was the first real cure of a mental illness in human history, and it had happened in another provincial outpost by an outcast psychiatrist, not in Paris or London. Not surprisingly, Cade's discovery failed to impress those in Paris and London, and he found it difficult to publish his findings in major psychiatric journals, ultimately publishing in the *Australia and New Zealand Journal of Psychiatry*, where they languished unread for a few years (Cade 1949). (In retrospect, Cade's 1949 discovery should have merited a Nobel Prize, as lithium has proven to be perhaps the most effective psychotropic treatment ever-the only agent proven to reduce death by suicide and to increase the life span and decrease overall mortality of persons with mental illness. Instead, that same year the last Nobel given for a psychiatric treatment was awarded for frontal lobotomy.)

Luckily, a young Swedish psychiatrist, Mogens Schou, whose brother had manic-depressive illness, saw the Australian report and took up the cause (Schou et al. 1954; Bech 2006). Schou had access to a new and unprecedented tool: randomized clinical trials (RCTs). The concept of randomization had been invented in the 1920s in agricultural research by statistician Ronald Fisher and had been applied to humans in medical research for the first time in 1948 (by British epidemiologist A. Bradford

Hill in a study of streptomycin for pneumonia; Stigler 1986). Schou applied the new method for the first time in psychiatry, simultaneously with others who used RCTs to study the first antipsychotic chlorpromazine, which had been discovered in 1952. Both sets of RCTs proved successful: lithium worked better than placebo for mania, and chlorpromazine worked better than placebo for schizophrenia (Healy 2001). Scientifically, the drugs had been proven in a manner that went far beyond all previous attempts at biological treatments in psychiatry. Clinically, psychiatrists saw dramatic improvement, not just marginal sedation or other symptomatic benefit, with these medications. In some cases, as with lithium, patients were literally cured and forever symptom free if they remained on the medication.

Within only a few years, chlorpromazine's use exploded, with millions of patients, especially in the crowded state hospitals, receiving the medication. But lithium floundered for about two decades, partly for political reasons. Chlorpromazine had been discovered in Paris by a pharmaceutical company, which obtained the support of Jean Delay, the powerful chairman of psychiatry at the main academic hospital, the Salpêtrière. From that base of power, chlorpromazine was marketed like soap flakes all across the world (Healy 2001).[2] Lithium, discovered by Cade in isolation and promoted by an unknown Swede, was an ion, available in rocks and streams, unpatented by any pharmaceutical company and therefore not marketed commercially. In the United States, it took two decades, until 1970, before the Food and Drug Administration approved lithium for medical use, and that approval came as the result of the efforts of academic psychiatrists, *not* the pharmaceutical industry.

By the 1970s, the psychopharmacology revolution was in full swing: lithium was prominently used for mania, chlorpromazine for schizophrenia, and antidepressants (tricyclics and monoamine oxidase inhibitors) for depression. While the psychoanalytic establishment could not ignore the rise of psychopharmacology, it could retort that psychopharmacology was purely symptom oriented. The psychoanalytic mainstream made the mistake of thinking that lithium was no different than bromides had been. In the nineteenth and early twentieth centuries, medications were used for mental illness as well, except medication treatment was purely symptomatic, not curative. For instance, bromides were simply sedatives; they could help calm a psychotic agitated person, but they did not markedly improve the episode of psychosis or alter the course of schizophrenia. Psychoanalysts thought lithium and imipramine were no different. But the claim made by the psychopharmacologists was different: they saw lithium, for instance, as cutting short a manic episode *and* as preventing all future mood episodes (Bech 2006). In effect, the drug cured the illness. Psychoanalysts could not integrate this possibility with their belief in purely superficial benefits of medications.

Psychoanalysts hoped that the psychopharmacology fad would blow over once everyone realized that these medications only mollified superficial symptoms but did not treat the underlying illness (which psychoanalysis presumably did). Time would prove psychoanalysts wrong, as indeed some of the new medications, like lithium, seemed to treat the overall disease entity and not just the symptoms. Perhaps more important, the domination of psychoanalysis was doomed to end due to the confluence of the two forces bubbling below the surface: the diagnostic and psychopharmacology revolutions.

The *DSM-III* Revolution

At the same time as lithium was finally marketed and clinicians gained more and more experience with chlorpromazine and imipramine, the Washington University school began to publish their studies validating Kraeplinian definitions of schizophrenia, bipolar disorder, and unipolar depression. It took little effort to connect the dots. The psychopharmacology revolution appeared to validate, and to make practical, the Kraepelinian paradigm, which had been derided for decades by Meyer and by psychoanalysts as being therapeutically useless. Lithium worked for bipolar disorder, imipramine for unipolar depression, and chlorpromazine for schizophrenia. Kraepelin had been vindicated; finally, in that grand struggle, Freud had to take a knee.

The great change occurred in 1980, not with the fanfare of a presidential election (such as that of Ronald Reagan) but with as much impact. In the late 1970s, the American Psychiatric Association had authorized a task force to update its diagnostic guidelines, the *Diagnostic and Statistical Manual* (*DSM*). This in itself was not unusual, as the *DSM* was updated about once a decade. It had first been written in 1952, with a second revision in 1968. The task itself did not seem particularly important to the psychoanalytic mainstream; they had by and large ignored the first two editions of the manual anyway. Those guidelines had little impact on a field that did not think psychiatric diagnosis was important. The diagnostic definitions in *DSM* were needed for the psychiatric administrators who kept the books in the mental hospitals and perhaps for the accountants who needed numbers for diagnoses in the insurance industry. *DSM* diagnoses were not scientifically or clinically useful. If they need to be revised for the administrators and accountants, so be it, they reasoned, but let us not put too much effort into it. As a consequence, when the American Psychiatric Association (APA) appointed the task force to revise the manual, it was populated by only those interested in the topic (which excluded the psychoanalysts) and headed by Robert Spitzer, a Ph.D. psychologist whose main interest was in diagnosis. Spitzer solicited the active involvement of the St. Louis group, which was the only research department focused on psychiatric diagnosis.

Under the radar, *DSM-III* was developed, a radical departure from the second edition, one in which Kraepelin's diagnostic concepts were largely resuscitated. Klerman, who had since moved to Cornell University in New York, also participated partly in the process, and he dubbed this new school that had developed as "neo-Kraepelinian" (Klerman 1986). Once *DSM-III* came out, psychoanalysts would complain about the undue influence of an "invisible college," meaning the St. Louis department and its collaborators, on the task force, yet this influence was largely due to the fact that the psychoanalytic leadership saw the whole process as unimportant until late in the process.

Near the end, when the task force's recommendations needed to be ratified by the APA leadership, the psychoanalytic establishment realized that *DSM-III* was a body blow in their struggle with the rising psychopharmacologists. Last-minute revisions were made: Dysthymia and generalized anxiety disorder, for instance, were added to incorporate the bread and butter of what paid the psychoanalysts' bills—"neurotic depression." The St. Louis school had wanted to include only major depression, excluding milder depressive and anxiety symptoms (Healy 1998). But it was too late.

DSM-III hit the field in 1980 like a tidal wave. The revolutionaries were no longer in the countryside; they had taken over the very government of psychiatry.

The Need for the Biopsychosocial Model

It was already happening, and *DSM-III* would speed the trend: psychiatrists everywhere were prescribing the new medications. For psychoanalysts, the stakes were high. How were they to preserve their approach and their way of life? Forced to cede some power to the psychopharmacologists, they needed to find a way to protect some of their territory.

Because recourse to the sacred writ of Freud's writings would no longer do, nor would any proposed authoritative interpretations by his heirs, Engel's writings began to attract major attention in psychiatry.

Criticism of the BPS model was rare. One of the few dissenters noted that there was a wish among mental health professionals to find a rationale for preserving the clinical use of psychotherapies, while also allowing the growing using of psychopharmacology:

> One of the major tasks facing contemporary psychiatry is finding a paradigm that retains the valuable contribution of psychoanalysis but that places it in the context of a more comprehensive account of mental illness. Such a paradigm must make sense of multiple etiologies and treatments, particularly the combined use of psychoactive drugs, individual dynamic therapy, behavior modification, and family, group, and milieu approaches. Obviously any model that meets these needs must not only be extremely broad but also define the appropriate domains of the various approaches. The leading candidate for the job is biopsychosocial eclecticism. This position maintains that psychiatric disorders have biological, psychological, and social determinants and that optimal treatment involves a combination of biological, psychological, and social interventions. (E. M. Abroms 1983)

Thus, a major raison d'être for the biopsychosocial model is to provide a justification for combined psychopharmacology-psychotherapy treatments. In the historical setting in which psychotherapy was the predominant treatment, the political role of the biopsychosocial model was to accept the inevitable rise of psychopharmacology, while seeking to prevent the demise of psychotherapies.[3]

Cease-fire

So we have one of those unique coincidences of history. In 1980, the same year that *DSM-III* was published—a de facto victory for psychopharmacologists in the war against psychoanalysis—Engel's key biopsychosocial model article was published-essentially a rejoinder to the biological psychiatry movement. Engel's model was certainly not as antipathetic to biological approaches as traditional psychoanalysis, so it was a compromise on the part of the psychoanalysts. Similarly, for biological psychiatrists, victory was never certain and fifty years of psychoanalysis had taken its toll. Major leaders like Klerman emphasized that they were not claiming that all problems in psychiatry were due to the brain and that psychoanalysis or psychotherapies had no role. The neo-Kraepelinians (unlike the Old Man himself) were willing to cede some territory to the psychoanalysts.

Sometimes, historical connections cannot be found in documents or even in stated ideas but rather in the silent influence of personality on personality (as William Osler once put it). The leading political figure that ushered *DSM-III* into being was Melvin Sabshin, the medical director of the APA (he is named on the dedication page of *DSM-III* as the guide to its coming into existence). Sabshin was a close disciple and student of Roy Grinker Sr. Perhaps it was not just a coincidence: maybe *DSM-III* and the rise of the BPS model are twins, the one reflecting the other.

A psychiatric Beirut was created. The psychopharmacologists now had some power; the psychoanalysts also had their own fiefdoms. The Green Line was patrolled by the biopsychosocial model, which was the cease-fire after a century of psychiatric wars between the mind and brain dogmas.

A curious thing has happened in the past three decades, however. Cease-fires are, by their nature, temporary instruments. They are a way to avoid further loss of life until some permanent new constitution or new power structure can be created. They are bandages, not solutions. Yet mental health professionals have come to believe that the biopsychosocial model, their cease-fire, has solved their problems. In reality, what worked well for a while in the 1980s began to fray in the 1990s and has begun to collapse entirely in the twenty-first century. Dissatisfaction is on the rise again.

The Pharmaceutical Industry Goblin

There are two pachyderms in this chapter on politics and psychiatry, as yet undiscussed: the pharmaceutical industry and the post-1980 evolution of the *DSM*s.

I will now touch the tusks of these elephants.

Many focus their distrust on biological dogmatism: they blame the pharmaceutical and insurance industries, and our compliance with them, for this state of affairs (Healy 1998). I do not disagree with the validity of these claims but reject their postmodernist tone: as if what has happened in psychiatry over the past two decades is *merely* about power and money and nothing else. I take ideas seriously, independent of their political or economic contexts. The pharmaceutical and insurance companies would never have been able to create "corporate psychiatry" if it was not for the intellectual emptiness of the BPS model. That is the Archimedean point: we can respond and change our current overreliance on drugs and our subservience to the whims of bureaucrats only if we have a coherent concept of psychiatry with which to fight back. The BPS model has failed in that role.

What about *DSM-IV* and *DSM-V*?

Has *The Diagnostic and Statistical Manual* evolved into better forms in its fourth revision of 1994 and its upcoming fifth revision planned for 2011? The writers of *DSM-III* can be faulted for many things, but at least they claimed that they wanted their faults to be critiqued and improved on in subsequent revisions. My observation is, though, that the APA leadership and those who have headed the revisions of *DSM-IV* and *DSM-V* tend toward a baseline conservatism: the threshold for making changes is set high, and little conceptual attention is paid to revising parts of the previous revision that have been disproven or no longer appear well grounded.

For all the political liberalism of mental health professionals, we are conceptually conservative.

I do not see *DSM-IV* or *DSM-V* as conceptually sound documents, nor do I see them as deeply flawed. If the *DSMs* are accepted and fit into the context of a method-based psychiatry, they can be useful and have some validity. When they are seen as the be-all, as in an uncritical evidence-based medicine (EBM) approach (see chapter 11), then they simply become expressions of biological dogmatism. Put another way, the manual can be used noneclectically in the interest of science and truth; it can also be used eclectically in a harmful manner. Like science itself, the editions of the *Diagnostic and Statistical Manual* are not inherently good or evil; their goodness or badness derives from how we use or abuse them.

Back from Politics

The cease-fire has only covered up smoldering tension that is rising to the surface again. Still, many refuse to acknowledge fact; the official view is that the current state of psychiatry is a culmination of a period of great progress that should continue uninterrupted in the morrow. It is time to honestly critique the biopsychosocial model, and while acknowledging its benefits, take stock of whether it is taking our field up to better havens or pulling it down into a mire of mediocrity.

Part II / The Fall of the Biopsychosocial Model

CHAPTER SEVEN

Drowning in Data

George Engel claimed that the biopsychosocial (BPS) model would provide a blueprint for research, yet the reality of the past two decades has not seemed to follow any particular blueprint.

Boundaryless Psychiatry

The most critical flaw of the biopsychosocial model is its eclecticism, which can be highlighted by asking the question: what are its boundaries? If we accept that the biopsychosocial model cannot simply be expanded forever without any boundaries, the question becomes when and how we are to put boundaries around it. Here is where the theory breaks down. As one critic put it (E. A. Abroms 1983): "Is it not true that in a given disorder one of the levels might provide the most important causal explanations and the other levels relatively less important ones? For example, is not manic-depressive disorder primarily an inherited biochemical disease and only secondarily and much less importantly a psychological and social problem? Are not the neuroses and personality disorders primarily psychosocially determined, reactive to environmental events, and biologically determined only to the extent that temperament is always influenced by constitution?"

Even if one accepts the BPS model and its basic premises, it is incomplete. It de-emphasizes, for instance, existential and spiritual approaches (at least in Engel's version). Engel's perspective, it must be recalled, was highly influenced by psychoanalysis, and many proponents of the biopsychosocial model continue to interpret the psychological component from the psychoanalytic perspective. While this need not be the case, and behavioral and other psychological theories can be used, existential or spiritual psychological approaches are infrequently used. The biopsychosocial model does not guide us as to which psychological theories are relevant.

Socially, one might take an interventional model with political commitments, as is often proposed by the social work discipline, or perhaps a more academic approach emphasizing life event correlates of illness, or maybe a public health approach looking at structural social factors (class, race, poverty) rather than individual ones. All these interpretations of the social aspect of the BPS model could be supported and again the model can be stretched in any direction.

One might take it even further: Long before Engel first described the BPS model in 1977, and apparently even before Roy Grinker's first use of the term *biopsychosocial* in 1952, existential psychiatrist Victor Frankl spoke of the "somatopsychospiritual" nature of humanity. Frankl argued that the biological approach of traditional psychiatry and the psychoanalytic approach of Freud need to be augmented by attention to spiritual aspects of humanity (in his existential method, which he called *logotherapy*; Frankl 1986). Engel and Grinker specifically excluded spiritual aspects from their model; but why? Why should one stop at psychology (and specifically psychoanalysis in the case of Engel) and not include spirituality?

One could then go even further: why stop at traditional spirituality? In the early 1990s, John Mack, a psychoanalyst at Harvard, well respected and a full professor on the psychiatry faculty, concluded that posttraumatic stress disorder was sometimes the result of alien abduction. His work on that topic produced a popular bestseller, though it was never published in scientifically respectable journals (Mack 2007). The BPS model could neither support nor stop Mack's speculations. When an eclectic theory is so boundaryless, what is to stop it from becoming not simply biopsychosocial, but biopsychosocial-intergalactic?

Where to start? Where to stop? The biopsychosocial model gives mental health professionals permission to do everything but no specific guidance to do anything. In an analogy suggested by Paul McHugh and Phillip Slavney (McHugh and Slavney 1998 [1983]), the biopsychosocial model is like a list of ingredients, as opposed to a recipe. To cook a meal, it is not sufficient to simply know the list of ingredients. One also needs to know how much of each ingredient one needs and in which order to add it. The biopsychosocial model lists relevant aspects of psychiatry but is silent as to how to understand those aspects in different conditions and in different circumstances (McLaren 1998).

Research and Reductionism

These features of the BPS model impair it as a guide to research, because success in medical research is predicated on the ability to focus. Medical research cannot be conducted in a general manner. One has to have specific hypotheses that are testable; the more specific, the more testable they tend to be. In advancing a research career, students do well to hone their skills on one small topic, on which they can become an expert. A biological researcher, for instance, may spend an entire career studying nothing but the axons of a particular species of snail. Or a medical researcher may focus his entire career on a subset of opiate receptors in the substantia gelatinosa of the spinal cord.

Scientific research is specific and focused. The BPS model is broad and vague. How can it be a blueprint for research?

It might be objected that this kind of super-specialization is in fact a major problem with medical research, emblematic of the biomedical reductionism that Engel fought. Yet, the question ought to be asked: is reductionism always wrong? In other words, if it turns out that diabetes partly involves specific abnormalities of subtypes of insulin receptors in the islets cells of Langerhans in the pancreas, is it wrong for someone to focus her research on those receptors?

The battle cry of antireductionism is often taken for granted, as if it is always and everywhere wrong to be reductionist. Here is an important fact: it is sometimes right and sometimes wrong to be reductionist. It depends on the problem or condition at hand (this, by the way, is a key difference between antieclectic method-based psychiatry and the BPS model; see chapter 16). The key question is determining when reductionism is justified and when it is not. The BPS model, at least in its most common usage, prejudges the matter, seeing reductionism as mostly useless.

Even Roy Grinker, perhaps the strongest psychiatric advocate of the BPS model, admitted the need for specificity in research (without specifically noting how it was a problem for the BPS approach): "One of the most serious problems in clinical research in psychiatry, in which so many variables exist and seem to cry out for consideration, is the tendency initially to include too much data, without focusing on the material meaningful to the particular problem. One cannot study everything at one time. It is necessary to be content with small parts of the total system, well-described subsystems, or pay the price of becoming inundated with indigestible numbers" (Grinker 1977).

When a Congressional committee is deciding how much funding to direct to the National Institute of Mental Health (NIMH), and NIMH leaders are deciding how to divvy up those funds among different psychiatric conditions, and when NIMH experts and consultants are deciding which specific research projects to fund—in short, in the real process of research funding, the BPS model provides no guidance as to how to direct those funds. Its blueprint is empty, for it dogmatically rejects reductionism.

The Biopsychosocial Model and Policy Making

NIMH consultants need to decide whether to fund this study on the glutamate receptor in schizophrenia as opposed to that study on family-oriented psychotherapy for schizophrenia. How are they to choose among those two studies? An adherent to the BPS model would view them as equally valid; the model provides no specific reason to lean one way or the other; it is up to the whim of the NIMH consultants or perhaps the winds of prevailing opinion on Capitol Hill. In fact, the leadership of NIMH has tended to take the view that biologically based studies should be given preference for funding, and psychiatric leaders, despite their fealty to the BPS model, have not successfully made the argument that funding should be directed toward psychological interventions. The BPS model has not been convincing, partly because it cannot explain why psychosocial research should be given more prominence than has been the case in schizophrenia, for instance. For if it is claimed that schizophrenia is partly biological, partly psychological, and partly social, the problem arises that a limited pot of funds needs to be distributed, and biological research seems to have produced a great deal more fruitful results than past psychosocial research.

Research in schizophrenia may be best directed in the biological direction, and in other conditions, such as posttraumatic stress disorder, it might be best directed in the psychosocial direction. Within each general category, research needs to be further directed to specific lines of investigation that appear most promising (for instance, glutamate research versus dopamine in schizophrenia, or neurotransmitter versus second messenger research in mood disorders, or cognitive behavioral versus psychoanalytically oriented therapy in posttraumatic stress disorder). In all these areas, more and more specific decisions need to be made, none of which receive any guidance from the highly general axioms of the BPS model. Far from being any kind of direct or efficient blueprint, the BPS approach is as useful to research as a map of the continents is useful to someone who wants to find the highways needed to drive from Atlanta to Washington.

Grinker on the Biopsychosocial Model and Research

In discussing research, Grinker, while eclectic and holistic elsewhere, acknowledged that BPS eclecticism was not helpful. After introducing the term *bio-psycho-social* as "encompassing all aspects of the living organism," he admits that "the term is not easy to grasp theoretically and difficult to implement operationally. With its holistic concepts it is often used to deny the significance of particular frames of reference and the importance of one or another variable in health or illness. I have little use for the futile plea to utilize holistic approaches operationally. The scientist has to focus, with a particular frame of reference and from a specified position, on a part of the world of man. Yet unified or holistic concepts in general are important as organizing principles for the understanding of general processes" (Grinker 1966). In other words, he advocated the BPS model as an overall theory of psychiatry but admitted its limited utility for guiding research—an astute observation.

Grinker also emphasized how dogmatic psychoanalysis had harmed research: "Psychoanalysis has seriously interfered with clinical research," he wrote. When psychoanalysts tried to contribute to nosology, "such abortions as 'passive-aggressive personality' have been induced" (Grinker 1966). Grinker avowed that the rise of psychopharmacology, the development of new drugs, had been the major spur to more clinical research in psychiatry, a development that he greeted happily. Elsewhere (Grinker 1969), he discussed the case of schizophrenia to highlight the dilemmas of research: many "little answers," which are difficult to integrate, are provided by clinical research. The student, trying to following those bits of data, arrives at "a point of redundancy of information or 'noise.'" The reason for this state of affairs is the biopsychosocial nature of mental illness; no single cause can be discovered for schizophrenia, only multiple factors. Grinker emphasized the interrelation between clinical and biological research, because "*what* is being studied," the clinical syndromes on which biological work is based, depends on clinical studies in nosology. The dilemma of reductionism versus holism was clear to him: "It is not that we should discard theories appropriate to various levels of organization and experience, nor abolish specific methods of investigation. To put each in an appropriate position within a total field, so that the transaction among its parts may be defined . . . presents a larger more correct view of any bio-psycho-social system. At the same time, it does not sacrifice the hard sciences of experimentation nor the softer sciences of behavioral observation" (Grinker 1969).

Model as "Meta-theory"

It might be argued that the BPS model provides a general rationale for research to proceed on all fronts, along with a strong argument for multidisciplinary research. In the general systems theory (GST) that underlies the BPS model, the idea is that any one level of knowledge is insufficient and that complete knowledge is obtained only by understanding a level of knowledge in the context of the whole system. Interactions between levels of knowledge become an important feature of understanding the system. Grinker, having been an active psychiatric researcher, viewed the BPS model as useful for research in this sense. He cites another researcher: "[GST] hopes to develop something like a 'spectrum' of theories—a system of systems which may perform the function of a 'gestalt' in the theoretical construction. Such 'gestalts' in special fields have been of great value in directing research toward the gaps which they reveal" (Grinker 1969).

Grinker admits the limits of GST (and by analogy the BPS model based on it):

> Theories serve heuristic purposes and are never meant to endure should they be shown to be internally inconsistent and fruitless in generating testable hypotheses. A theory of systems should do more than furnish satisfaction for believers as if it were a religion. General systems theory has had its share of criticism on this score. . . . One critic asks the question "So what? It only establishes analogies among levels of organization or a number of systems and contributes no real progress." Yet, analogies are indeed significant sources from which to create new approaches to problem areas. . . . General systems theory has no methodology, as do no other theories, but it does establish a paradigm or outline a way of thinking of relationships, of parts and wholes. (Grinker 1969)

Here Grinker states that indeed the GST (and I would add the BPS model) does not have a specific methodology and thus is not a direct guide for research. He argues that it can serve, however, as a "meta-theory" that might highlight directions in which research must go. Grinker errs in claiming that no theory has a methodology. An antieclectic, pluralist, method-based model of psychiatry, such as the work of Karl Jaspers (chapters 15–17), is all about methods and nothing but methods and thus is much more useful for guiding research. The biopsychosocial model and general systems theory eschew methods and function at the level of general and vague analogies. While this can be useful to some extent, as Grinker admits, it is hardly a robust blueprint for research: "Are we able to utilize general systems theory in all our clinical investigations by extracting hypotheses subject to observational or experimental proof? The answer is 'no.' Rarely, if at all, are we able to use the total theory or to even envisage total wholeness. Although we are able to define some special structures . . . we still must limit ourselves to parts of systems, or, better said, to small systems. But we can, indeed, know where we are in perceived reality. . . . In most investigations general systems theory has limited practicability, depending on the research focus" (Grinker 1969).

Certainly the biopsychosocial model and the general systems theory would support an emphasis on multidisciplinary research, with researchers specializing in one field communicating with those in other fields, but again the BPS model does not provide specificity of when and how these kinds of interactions should occur. It can be viewed as simply supporting such multidisciplinary work in general, in all circumstances, but this viewpoint is not useful for government agencies making decisions about how to allocate funding or for specific researchers making decisions on how to investigate certain topics.

The Science of the Art of Medicine

One of the rare places in which proponents of the BPS model have addressed the question of research directly is in an edited book by colleagues and students of Engel (Frankel, Quill, and McDaniel 2003). In a chapter on research entitled "The Science of the Art of Medicine," the authors (G. C. Williams et al. 2003) associate the BPS approach with "humanizing medicine" (or the "patient-centered approach," which Engel arguably deemphasized in his wish to be seen as scientific and not simply humanistic; see next chapter). At the University of Rochester, Engel founded the Program for Biopsychosocial Studies, the content of which was defined as involving psychoneuroimmunology, "systematic desensitization for chemotherapy patients," "in-depth longitudinal case studies of patient experiences," and the association of the physician-patient relationship to medical outcomes. Engel's colleagues also discussed the relevance of other fields of research, especially family systems theory and self-determination theory in psychology, as allied to the BPS approach, and they connect gene-environment interaction with the BPS perspective. Perhaps this nonexhaustive list more or less identifies the scope of research in which the BPS model has been, and can be, applied. One need hardly remark how vast a field of research is left untouched by these applications.

The Healing Context

Another attempt to understand the relevance of the BPS for research can be made by returning to the U.K. conference on the BPS model that was reviewed in chapter 5 (White 2005). The main discussion of research at that conference involved a study of the "healing process and context in randomized controlled trials" (Kleijnen 2005). The author discussed the nonspecific factors involved in placebo-related improvement, as well as such contextual factors as how researchers spoke with participants in the study and even how drugs were administered and the color of the pills given. In the discussion, the chairman of the conference made some respectful but critical comments: "You have actually taken us further in the BPS model than from where we began. I was expecting you to end up with a review of how brilliant cognitive behaviour therapy is and how fantastic models based on the BPS model are. In fact, you have gone even beyond this to genuinely 'touchy-feely' qualities in clinical interactions. On the way, did you go through interventions that explicitly use the BPS model as opposed to what you have done, which is to look at the nontangible factors of clinical interactions?" (White 2005).

The presenter demurred. The chairman persisted: "There is a view that the explicit models of BPS interventions are not touchy-feely; that in themselves they are rigorous and have a theoretical basis. They are based on a certain model of how the body and mind interact, which they then seek to alter, as opposed to yours which are at most dealing with metaphysical qualities. You are attempting to measure the unmeasurable" (White 2005).

Later, another attendee expressed some dissatisfaction with how the topic of the BPS model and research had been addressed:

> As the discussion continues, I am getting increasingly confused. I naively thought the BPS model tried to address the inadequacies of the biomedical model because that focused solely on disease and treated human beings as machines. I thought the BPS model was trying to reintroduce both mind and body and operationalize that into social, psychological, and biological issues. But after we got the history and philosophy out of the way this morning, almost the whole of the rest of the day seems to me to have been trying to force social and psychological factors back into a proper biomedical model. It has been about psychological

and social factors to disease. I was beginning to be encouraged by [this] . . . paper, which was talking about expectations and people . . . [but then the chairman suggested] that we should forget about all this ethereal nonsense and get back to medicine. Since about 11 this morning, no one has mentioned the mind! (White 2005)

Even in the hands of its proponents, it is not clear if and how the BPS model is to be applied to research.[1]

Directionless Research

The consequence of the general irrelevance of the BPS model to research has been that research has proceeded without it, on its own, without any general theoretical orientation or blueprint. Some would say this is good, and in an ideal world—where research funds, time, research participants, and researchers were unlimited in supply—that might be the case. But in reality, hard decisions have to be made about what to study and why. These decisions are currently being made by individual researchers, based on their own specific theories or preferences. Hence studies come in all varieties; combined with the professional need to publish articles to survive in academia, psychiatry is now drowning in data but has no overarching way to put the available data together.

A corollary of this lack of utility of the BPS model for research has been a general skepticism about any kind of conceptual or theoretical writing in the psychiatric scientific literature. One can easily publish the 2,563rd article on a small sample of patients treated with a given drug, but it is well-nigh impossible to publish a conceptual article (such as, for instance, an article on the limits of the BPS model).

A general theory of psychiatry is probably unnecessary, unless one wants to go back to one of the two dogmas of psychiatry; yet multiple theories of psychiatry might be useful, if they could be targeted to specific conditions or justified in specific circumstances. The BPS model is the worst of both worlds: it is a single theory that teaches us little and provides no direction as multiple specific theories might.

We are left with a great deal of empirical data, but no general way of putting the data together, certainly not in that meta-theory sense that Grinker described. For the average mental health professional, not to mention psychiatric residents or medical students or the lay public, it is almost impossible to succinctly describe the nature of psychiatry or to explain scientifically based views of contemporary psychiatry on major psychiatric syndromes.

This lack of general orientation leads us to the next failure of the BPS model—its inability to serve as an orienting conceptual structure for psychiatric education.

CHAPTER EIGHT

Teaching Eclecticism

In a 1980 retirement Festschrift, George Engel's colleagues and former students emphasized that teaching was the most important aspect of his professional life (Ader and Schmale 1980). If the model was to shine anywhere, it should shine here.

Instead, in many settings, the biopsychosocial model has not served well in teaching medical students and psychiatric residents. Although it might be presented in a more nuanced way, one sometimes observes, even in prominent academic centers, relatively simplistic scenarios in which a case will be presented, and the teacher will ask the students to describe the case in three facets: bio, psycho, and social. Often, two of the facets are weakly explored, and the student, for whatever reason, leans toward one particular aspect of the case. Or, alternatively, no facet is explored in any depth.

Proponents of the BPS model might object that in their institution they may do a better job, and this may in fact be the case. It is not irrelevant, however, that the model can be, and often is, simplistically interpreted such that one only attains a relatively superficial understanding of a case. My suggestion is that this is not completely a fault of a poor use of the BPS approach but rather a consequence of the overinclusiveness of the model and its poor boundaries.

Engel on Education

Let us see what Engel himself had to say about how the BPS model could be used for medical education (G. L. Engel 1978). He describes how physicians using the biomedical model are often seen as "insensitive, callous, neglectful, arrogant, mechanical." He blames Descartes for this state of affairs (there seems to be no end to the horrors of dualism). He claims that diseases are dynamic processes, not discrete entities with causes. The psychosocial aspects of illness are ignored by biomedicine, seen as neither accessible to scientific scrutiny nor essential for medical education. This leads to the shotgun use of laboratory and diagnostic procedures, resulting in patients feeling "used, abused, and dehumanized." The laboratory tests sometimes say "no disease" yet the stubborn patient persists in feeling ill. (I recall an elderly hospitalized woman who looked pale and was less responsive verbally, yet her vital signs and blood tests results were mostly normal; the head nurse said, "Her numbers look better than she does." She was in the midst of a stroke and died within six hours.)

Engel does not claim that there is no role for reductionistic biomedicine but rather that it has become degraded from a once fruitful approach into a dogma. The leaders of biomedicine have responded to "public dissatisfaction" with the dehumanizing practice of medicine by turning to "a curiously regressive romanticism" and recommending "a sentimental return to the past" (G. L. Engel 1978). (Engel sets himself up as unsentimental and nonromantic.) Such educators recommend exposing medical students to practitioners earlier in their training and other such measures. What they ignore, Engel says, is "apply[ing] the scientific method to the human dimensions of medicine. The picture naively conjured up is that the scientific competence of today's physician can be blended with the legendary warmth, compassion, and common sense of the kindly family doctor of yesteryear." He dismisses this view as "false and devoid of logic," based on an overly romanticized view of the past; physicians were not more compassionate or humane in the past than they are now. The biomedical response, then, is to retreat to unscientific talk about the "art" of medicine, "based on intuition, professional rules, aphorisms, and maxims from the accumulated wisdom of experienced clinicians. . . . Nothing more than compassion, a humane attitude, and good common sense are needed" (G. L. Engel 1978). Most of these tasks can be delegated to other health professionals, such as nurses and social workers, Engel continues, leaving doctors free to do the hard work of biological diagnosis and treatment. With the biopsychosocial illness thus split up, adversarial relationships develop between nurses (or other health professionals) and doctors, leading to unnecessary professional conflict.

Engel wants to be more scientific. There is a science, he says, that is being neglected: the sciences of psychology and psychiatry and sociology and social work that can underlie scientifically based approaches to the psychosocial aspects of illness. The key, he argues, involves four essential attributes of all health care professionals (whether doctors or nurses or others): collaboration, communication, complementarity, and competence. Besides a fondness for the third letter of the alphabet, perhaps the most important feature of Engel's view here is that he is claiming that a biopsychosocial education about illness is not only more practical and more humane but also more scientific, appearances to the contrary. Perhaps the factor of competence has received the least attention in discussion of Engel's model. He himself puts it this way: "How stubborn and pernicious the influence of biomedical dogma can be is betrayed by those who say, 'I fully agree with your position but, when I get sick, I would rather have for my physician one who is conversant with the most up-to-date biomedical knowledge and techniques than one who understands my psyche'" (G. L. Engel 1978). Engel blames Descartes again: "Again dualism intrudes, as though competence in one sphere precludes competence in the other. The proper distinction is between a general level of competence and specialized competencies. . . . What is generally lacking now is the requirement that general competency include the psychosocial sphere. Current biomedical dogma designates psychosocial knowledge and skills a special competency, training for which is expected only of psychiatrists and other mental health professionals" (G. L. Engel 1978).

Engel goes on to make a distinction that conflicts with the views of those psychiatrists (Gabbard and Kay 2001) who claim that MD-psychiatrists are especially more competent than other mental health professionals because only MD-psychiatrists can have enough competence in all aspects of biopsychosocial illnesses: "For some tasks, any health professional, regardless of discipline, might be competent, while for other more specialized or complex tasks, only a professional with the knowledge and skills need for that particular task would be qualified, be it a speech therapist, a surgeon, a nutritionist, a nurse, or a psychiatric social worker" (G. L. Engel 1978).

Engel's summary forms the basis of the U.S. psychiatric oral board examinations today: "*All three levels,* biological, psychological, and social, must be taken into account *in every health care task*" (G. L. Engel 1978, italics added).[1] Every case must incorporate discussion of all three aspects.

Here, then, Engel lays out the basic theory of biopsychosocial education: All three aspects are relevant in all cases. No single illness or patient or condition can be reduced to any one aspect. They are all, more or less equally, relevant, in all cases, at all times.

Teaching Medical Students

Medical students are a special group for whom the BPS model does not rise to the educational task. Often the toughest audience, they are uncommitted to learning a trade (unlike psychiatry residents) and want data to support all arguments. For them, the choice of emphasizing one or the other aspect of the BPS model in a specific case can seem irrational or nonscientific. In an age in which psychoanalysis predominated, a psychoanalytic emphasis was preferred. Now, when psychopharmacology approaches have gained sway, biological emphases are often given. As philosopher George Santayana once said, in the United States, "ideas are abandoned in virtue of a mere change of feeling, without any new evidence or new arguments. We do not nowadays refute our predecessors, we pleasantly bid them goodbye" (Santayana 1924). Given that fewer medical students enter psychiatry (now only about 2%, one-half the number who entered two decades ago; Stock et al. 2006), it is possible that the limitations of the BPS model have contributed to this state of affairs.

Neither biological nor psychoanalytic dogmatisms appeal to medical students. If psychiatry is to be purely biological, many students will prefer to choose neurology as a specialty. If psychiatry is seen as purely psychoanalytic, it often fails to appeal to the scientific-mindedness of medical students as well. Medical students are either discouraged by the two dogmas of psychiatry or simply baffled by the vagueness of the BPS model.

Teaching at Engel's Institution

The experience of teaching this model in medical school at the University of Rochester is most informative, for difficulties there, where Engel had the most impact, would portend poorly for its use elsewhere.

In the 1980s, at the height of Engel's institutional influence there, the BPS model was incorporated in Rochester primarily in the first two years of medical school, with John Romano teaching a first-year course called Fundamental Concepts of Human Behavior and Engel teaching a second-year course called Psychopathology

(Brown 2003). Weekly conferences were also conducted in which patients told their stories and faculty commented on the cases from the biopsychosocial perspective. A program in medical humanities also provided exposure to cultural and humanistic aspects of medicine. A great deal of curriculum time was given to the BPS model, but both faculty and students were dissatisfied. The BPS model was emphasized in the preclinical years, in the fancy carpeted medical school halls; in the clinical years of grunt work on the hospital's tiled floors, it seemed less relevant: "BPS ends where the carpet ends," a medical student maxim went (Dannefer, Hundert, and Henson 2003). This was exemplified when a third year medical student in the 1990s asked, before oral examination of clinical skills: "Do you want me to do a BPS interview or a 'real' interview?" As Rochester faculty noted, "Students tended to associate BPS medicine with 'warm and fuzzy' communication skills taught in the first two years, decontextualized from 'real' clinical work of making a diagnosis and treating real patients who were often seriously ill. . . . Faculty were also expressing concern that the 'bio' was being taken out of the BPS. The curricular structure was faulted for the reduction of BPS medicine to 'communication skills'" (Dannefer, Hundert, and Henson 2003). Another example is found in an examination of letters written to Engel by former students: "In hindsight, one of the strange things is that there was a lot of talk about the Biopsychosocial Model. . . . It was a flag that people waved. And yet when you looked around to see where it was, it didn't exist. And when we got to the floors, in the third year, I'll always remember this, that one of the professors said, 'You guys have been taught all this BPS stuff. Now you're on the floors. You just forget all that.' . . . So, there were people who were waving a flag, who, if you came over, they had no country" (Dombeck et al. 2003). The leaders of the University of Rochester program saw the problem as one of failure to integrate theory and practice; they brought in a new dean and introduced a new curriculum that sought to incorporate BPS teaching more seamlessly throughout all four years of medical school (Dannefer, Hundert, and Henson 2003). The new approach has no follow-up as of yet; it could be that the problem may not simply be a generic one of failure to integrate theory and practice but rather a specific one, of this particular theory—the BPS model—not having much to offer in actual practice.[2]

The Biopsychosocial Model and Humanism

Engel's colleagues collected and examined, with his assistance, years of written correspondence with his former students, as a way of understanding the educational value of the BPS approach (Dombeck et al. 2003). In a nice piece of qualitative research, they concluded that a key theme was that "the BPS approach represented a way to treat a complete human being by focusing on the relationship between the patient and the physician." While admirable, as discussed in chapter 12, it is unclear what is special about the BPS model in this respect, as opposed to other humanistic approaches to medicine (such as Oslerian biomedicine). Other themes in this collection of essays were that the BPS model connected physical with psychological and social aspects of illness and that it focused on the physician-patient relationship, but these themes also are not unique to this approach.

Clearly his students viewed Engel's model as a variant on holistic or humanistic medicine. In their letters, former students used the words "humanistic" and "holistic" together frequently. One spoke of the need to achieve an "integration of humanism plus hypertechnology" (Dombeck et al. 2003). The equivalence of the BPS model with humanism was a constant impression on former students. One student commented on the liberating effect of attention to psychosocial material as scientifically important: "He [Engel] encouraged me to be scientific about whatever! He said, 'anything you can observe you can be scientific about,' and that one statement set me free." This former student had accepted Engel's insistence that the BPS model was scientific, in fact more scientific than the biomedical model, because "to be scientific in one's practice of medicine one needs to be curious about everything about the patient, including psychosocial data" (Dombeck et al. 2003).

All this emphasis on humanism as a vital aspect of the BPS approach in Rochester ignores the ironic fact that Engel wanted to banish all talk of humanism and the "art" of medicine, replacing it with the sciences of psychology and social factors (see below).

The educational core of the BPS model appears to be the claim that the physical aspects of illness need to be augmented by attention to the psychological and social. The emphasis on the importance of the clinical interview grows out of the less-unique components of the BPS model (i.e., the attention to the physician-patient relationship and the Oslerian emphasis on the person as opposed to simply the disease).

Grinker on Psychiatric Education

From Engel, we now turn to Roy Grinker's views on the BPS approach to psychiatric education. In a 1952 lecture (published four decades later; R. Grinker Sr. 1994), Grinker noted that "no one can imagine the future." He emphasized how a good psychiatrist needed to be a good physician, with four qualities: the ability to communicate with others, the ability to be self-corrective, an integrative capacity (able to stand up to stress), and strong ethics. Communication was the essence of psychiatry, he said, which he segued into his eclectic view of the importance of the biopsychosocial view and the multidisciplinary knowledge at the intersections of perspectives. He elsewhere emphasized three attitudes that need to be fostered in psychiatry residency: a spirit of investigation, a tolerance for aberrant ideas, and skepticism and scrutiny of what seems to be true (Grinker 1969).

On another occasion, a commentator on Grinker's paper "A Struggle for Eclecticism" (Grinker 1964) noted that psychiatric training programs were already struggling with how to be able to teach content while not being dogmatic. By broadening the residency experience to include many different approaches, one risked producing a "confusing smorgasbord" that would leave residents disoriented. How one would seek to organize faculties in an eclectic program was also of concern: If the faculty consisted of persons committed to different views, then there would be a "cold war of vying ideologies." If the faculty was chosen to represent "middle of the road" attitudes, then residents would be exposed to no one with any strong views about anything. Grinker responded by noting that in his program the emphasis was on exposing residents to as many different perspectives as possible; thus residents had about eighteen supervisors during three years of training, with each supervisor changing every six months. Elsewhere (Grinker 1965), he noted that education must not be reduced to "technical training" and that we must "educate disciplined investigators" who are committed to testing, not afraid to discard ideas, and imbued with a healthy skepticism.

If we accept Grinker's perspective, it is worth asking whether psychiatric training programs—or psychology or social work programs—are producing professionals who are skeptical about the biopsychosocial model. In fact, critique of the model is rare; it is frequently simply accepted as self-evident.

Teaching Psychotherapy

How can one be eclectic and still teach different methods more than superficially? In practice, most clinical psychology programs have a predominant orientation, often cognitive behavioral, sometimes still psychoanalytic: "Most therapists are still trained in one approach, and then gradually incorporate parts of other approaches once they discover the limitations of their original approach" (Norcross, Karpiak, and Lister 2005).

Arnold Lazarus provides an amusing anecdote on the limits of psychology training (Lazarus 1990): he describes a charismatic and interpersonally gifted friend, a dentist, who was so empathic and attractive to others that everyone said that he should have been a psychologist and in fact he seemed to provide a kind of psychotherapy to his dental patients. Lazarus himself confided in his dentist-friend with much benefit and advised others to seek counsel with him rather than with a professional therapist. Eventually, his friend began taking graduate courses in psychology and quipped: "Now when a patient comes to me I ask 'Is your problem mental or dental?' " Lazarus described the effect of formal psychology education on his friend: "As my friend learned more and more psychology . . . it seemed to me that his natural skills eroded. I have not forgotten the shock I felt when, shortly after my mother had died, I was opening my heart to him, to this naturally great therapist. . . . Instead of the deep understanding, support, empathy, and basic caring that I had come to expect, I received a string of platitudes and labels. . . . In my estimation, he never regained those special and natural relationship skills. . . . I continue to regard him as a prime example of someone who remains mutilated by his training and attendant superstitions." He went on to make the point that much of psychiatry and psychology residency training involves teaching people to behave less like naturally caring human beings and more within certain theoretical paradigms. He suggests that most of that teaching is simply false: "My teachers handed me a long list of do's and don'ts—actually more don'ts than do's. I think I have broken all the rules with excellent results." He goes on to note that there are, of course, some absolute don'ts, like having sex with patients. But the general point remains that most of the rules are simply dogmas that in fact are unproven or false.

How should one provide supervision in such a setting? If supervisors are dogmatists, they often give strong negative feedback when the trainee works outside prevailing doctrine. Being eclectic, Lazarus says he tries to provide his students "with various options, without labeling them correct or incorrect. I don't think we can argue too strongly for humility and tentativeness given the current state of our basic knowledge. Organic medicine has a 300-year jump on us" (Lazarus 1990). The problem is: how can you teach anything if you are unsure of what to teach?

A Thought Experiment

Let us suppose that I have a 35-year-old patient who has manic-depressive illness; his father had it, and his father, and six cousins, and twelve aunts and uncles. Suicides occurred in the family every generation for six generations running. The patient's illness began at age 19 with a manic episode, which resolved in four months, followed by depression and one mania yearly, alternating with two to three years of wellness. The depressive periods tend to last six months and are associated with notable suicidality at times; two attempts led to hospitalization. The patient notes that he is different when manic and depressed, but he says he cannot control himself. Most episodes occur in the setting of some kind of stress or life event, one depression happened after a child was born, another after an aunt got sick, another after his divorce; a manic episode began after he started a new job, another after he lost one. In sum, this patient is a walking textbook case of Kraepelinian manic-depressive illness. Here is the question: what would the biopsychosocial model suggest be done and what would the biomedical model suggest?

The year is 1978. Lithium has been available in the United States for eight years, yet most American psychiatrists are not biologically oriented. The BPS consultant would be in the mainstream, the biological consultant in the minority. Here is the imaginary discussion:

> BPS CONSULTANT: Well, in this case, we need to pay attention to biological, psychological, and social components of this patient's illness, components that are so interwoven as to be impossible to separate. Obviously, a strong genetic component makes this patient susceptible to manic or depressive episodes; unfortunately, genetics are not amenable to change. Biologically, there may be a mechanism, as yet unknown, in the brain that leads to the presentation of his symptoms. Psychologically, there is a great deal of affective response to losses in life as well as to its challenges. This extreme nature of affective response may have some origins in childhood, perhaps too-distant parents, perhaps repeated frustration in getting what he wanted at the breast or in later development. We do not know the exact nature of his early childhood and important parental relationships; these will need to be explored. Socially, this patient is having a great deal of difficulty with the two great tasks of life: to love and to work. These problems are exacerbating his constitutional predispositions to flee into mania or to wallow in depression. Attention to the nature of those relationships and his ability to navigate the real world of work and marriage will also be important.
>
> I recommend daily psychoanalysis. As an adjunct, purely for symptom control, you can also prescribe benzodiazepines for sleep, imipramine for depressive symptoms, or thioridazine when manic symptoms are out of control. But I doubt he will get better until he has experienced a few years of hard work in dynamic psychotherapy.

THE BIOLOGICAL CONSULTANT: This is a biological disease of the brain of mostly genetic origin with a likely biochemical cause to be discovered. We know, in the meantime, that lithium is effective in preventing both manic and depressive episodes. Give lithium.

Which is the better approach?

Here is the same discussion in 2006. Now the roles are reversed: the biological approach to psychiatry is more prominent, the psychoanalytic in retreat, the cognitive behavioral model in advance, and the BPS model nominally accepted but in practice poorly understood.

BPS CONSULTANT: Well, in this case, we need to pay attention to biological, psychological, and social components of this patient's illness, components that are so interwoven as to be impossible to separate. Obviously, a strong genetic component makes this patient susceptible to manic or depressive episodes; unfortunately, genetics are not amenable to change. Biologically, the brain mediates the expression of his symptoms. Pharmacologically, mood stabilizers such as lithium have been shown to be helpful. Psychologically, the patient may be responding to life stresses with negative thinking patterns that exacerbate his problems, sending him further into depression. Socially, immediate triggers of his episodes are important, such as poor sleep habits, excessive activity at nighttime, and conflict in his interpersonal relationships due to poor developmental interpersonal skills that likely result from years of the disruptive effects of his mood episodes in his life. I recommend lithium for the manic symptoms and Prozac for the depressive symptoms, because they are more prominent, and individual cognitive behavioral therapy for the depressive component, along with group therapy to assist with his interpersonal skills.

THE BIOLOGICAL CONSULTANT: This is a biological disease of the brain of mostly genetic origin with a likely biochemical cause to be discovered. We know, in the meantime, that lithium and other mood stabilizers are effective in preventing both manic and depressive episodes. Give lithium.

Now obviously in both eras, the biological consultant could have added psychotherapies as adjuncts to lithium, but I have kept it simple. The issue is whether one gains much in the way of added benefit with the BPS approach beyond simply using lithium, an effective medication by itself for this condition. (I am not suggesting that added psychosocial interventions may not aid lithium; I am suggesting that their marginal benefit in this case may not be large.)

Clearly, the BPS approach in the 1970s was off the mark: equal attention to all three components is irrelevant in this condition. A modernized BPS model might be more valid, because at least it includes the effective treatment, but it also includes much else that may be unnecessary or poorly proven (generic group therapy) or even harmful (antidepressant medications, which can cause mania when given in a symptom-based approach to treatment).

Engel's Antihumanism

Perhaps the bottom line of the educational benefit of the BPS approach, as it was proposed by Engel and continues to be emphasized by its current psychiatric proponents, is to seek to avoid biological reductionism. Good enough. Yet this can be done in multiple other ways. For instance, William Osler put even more effort into medical education than did Engel (see chapter 12). We can view the two as proposing opposing models for medical practice and education. Osler proposed the biomedical model, leavened by the humanities (seen as the arts and not some variety of psychological science). Engel proposed the BPS model, with no need for the humanities, using psychosocial perspectives based on the sciences of psychology, psychiatry, sociology, and public health. The particular scientific views Engel used, often derived from psychoanalysis, were not scientifically proven in any way that is currently justifiable. Rather, they were psychological ideologies masquerading as science. Abstracting from that historical reality, is there any advantage to legislating away the humanities and insisting on scientific use of psychology and sociology in addition to our biomedical approach? The difficulty with the BPS model in education has been that sometimes the psychosocial components appear to be relevant to understanding medical cases or conditions and sometimes they do not, yet the BPS approach seems to imply that they are always relevant; or if not, it fails to provide us guidance as to when they are relevant and when they are not. A humanistic approach to every patient is always relevant, and, if we are in fact limiting our discussion to diseases, the biological component is always relevant. To that extent, as will be explained in more detail in chapter 12, Osler got it much more right than Engel.

The only mildly critical voice at Engel's retirement Festschrift (Ader and Schmale 1980) came from one of the few speakers who had been a colleague, not a student, of Engel. Speaking of efforts to introduce psychiatric consultation to general medical wards, the author wrote: "I knew . . . that we could not just graft on a psychiatric model. We had to see illness as a human event. Such a conviction appears to be shared by all contributors to this Festschrift. They're singing: 'For he's a jolly good fellow.' Couldn't we replace that complex term: biopsychosocial, with the *human* variable? I'm going to one-up you. I'm saddened that every time I use the term human it reminds my medical peers of corrupted humanistic or holistic practices and they visualize a host of swamis swarming over the campus." The swami nightmare was the same one that disturbed von Bertalanffy's REM sleep (von Bertalanffy 1974) and that Grinker repeatedly disparaged (Grinker 1964, 1970). Perhaps the BPS model can be seen as a 1960s-era bourgeois reaction to that kind of countercultural humanism: Look, it said, we'll introduce the human variable, but let's do it scientifically (buttoned-up) rather than culturally (with bell bottoms). But the 1960s are over.

The purpose of professional education in psychiatry or psychology or medicine is to prepare students for real-world practice (see Appendix). The next step in our analysis of the claims of the BPS model is to move from its role in teaching to students to its role in guiding the actual practice of psychiatrists, mental health professionals, and physicians. Medical education was supposed to be the strong suit of the BPS model; yet we found it wanting in a number of ways. Actual clinical practice, we will see, is where its failures appear even more prominent.

CHAPTER NINE

Psychopharmacology Awry

In diseases of the mind . . . it is an art of no little importance to adminis-
ter medicines properly; but, it is an art of much greater importance and
more difficult acquisition to know when to suspend or altogether to
omit them.   PHILLIPPE PINEL, *A TREATISE ON INSANITY*, 1806

The next test is whether the biopsychosocial (BPS) model meets George Engel's
criterion as "a design for action." Previously, I discussed how the model has been,
and continues to be, a means of preserving a space for psychotherapies; yet few
would claim success there. Less noticed than this, it also has failed to provide psychiatry with a rational grounding for the practice of psychopharmacology. This
matter is relevant because most psychiatrists today practice psychopharmacology,
not psychotherapies, and thus one would want the main theory of psychiatry to
have some relevance to that practice.

It might be objected that I am asking for a philosophy of psychopharmacology.
Why should psychopharmacology need a philosophy? Should it not stand on its
own, based on its own data? Such questions usually come from those who either
have no experience with scientific research or from researchers with a simplistic
notion of science. It is now widely accepted in the philosophy of science, and in statistical theory, that data never speak for themselves: they always need to be interpreted.[1] In the process of interpreting them one uses conceptual assumptions that
exist outside of the data. In the application of data to practice, numerous conceptual assumptions are in play. An honest examination of the nature of science would

lead us to conclude that scientists too have conceptual assumptions—philoso-phies—that influence them. Similarly, practicing psychiatrists have a philosophy of psychopharmacology; it is time to assess it.

Eclectic Psychopharmacology

It might also be objected that the BPS model never claimed to provide conceptual backing for psychopharmacology. Yet a reading of Engel's work demonstrates that he viewed it as a broad *scientific* model that encompasses all of medicine, not just a part of it. The point is not simply to apply it to psychosocial issues but to all of medicine, including biological aspects, such as psychopharmacology.

A skeptic might finally say that the implication of the BPS approach for psycho-pharmacology is simply that it should not be applied reductionistically, alone, without also incorporating psychosocial interventions. I will take up this issue in the next chapter, yet even if one allows for this interpretation, the key question is how this view of the BPS model influences our understanding of the nature of psy-chopharmacology treatment per se.

Paul McHugh, former chair of the Department of Psychiatry at the Johns Hop-kins University, once published an influential article, later included in his book *The Mind Has Mountains,* about psychoanalytic excesses that led to the suicide of a Harvard medical student entitled "Psychotherapy Awry" (McHugh 2006). Now let us look at *psychopharmacology awry.*

Non-Hippocratic Psychopharmacology

Medicine is (or should be) all about diagnosis, followed by treatment. Without a diagnosis, treatments are generally less effective, only symptomatic, and often bet-ter avoided. This is the Hippocratic approach to medicine, a viewpoint known by most physicians only as a label but not in its content (Ghaemi 2008). If we truly ac-cept this tradition, then psychopharmacology should be primarily about diagno-sis and only secondarily about pharmacology. In other words, the hardest part of psychopharmacology practice is determining what diagnosis the patient has (or does not have), not the details of the effects of medications or which medications to choose. Once we have the diagnosis right, then we know which medications to choose; if indeed a disease is present and we have effective medications for it, then treatment usually can proceed with little difficulty.

The main mistake I see among psychiatrists today is that they are sloppy in diagnosis; diagnoses are matters of indifference, and people are treated for symptoms. For depressive symptoms, psychiatrists prescribe antidepressants; for insomnia, sedatives; for anxiety, anxiolytics; for cognitive problems, amphetamines; for mood swings, mood stabilizers; and for unusual thoughts or erratic or aggressive behavior, antipsychotics. Many practitioners even think it best to "cover all their bases": because most patients have some anxiety and depressive symptoms along with unusual behavior, they often end up taking an antidepressant, an anxiolytic, and an antipsychotic. This "cocktail" is purely symptom based, completely unscientific, and frequent; indeed nonmedical critics are right that almost anyone could practice this kind of psychopharmacology which leads to more harm than good.[2]

Many psychiatrists may object to this description, so let me spell out the reasons for the inadequacy of this approach.

Failed Treatment Means Incurable Disease

In the era of psychoanalytic dogmatism, psychoanalysis was prescribed for almost any psychiatric condition, including even schizophrenia. When some conditions, such as psychosis, appeared resistant to psychoanalysis, these syndromes were reformulated to agree with psychoanalytic theory, rather than vice versa. Thus, for instance, in the 1950s, the concept of "pseudoneurotic schizophrenia" became popular, defined as those persons who came to psychoanalysis with neurotic symptoms and yet, when put on the couch, became even more ill, exhibiting psychotic symptoms *as a result of psychoanalysis* (never having been psychotic spontaneously). Instead of viewing psychoanalysis as harmful, the psychoanalysts blamed the patients: they had an illness that made them prone to such reactions. The solution: more psychoanalysis, with some variations in technique. The illness was relabeled "borderline personality organization" in the late 1960s and entered *The Diagnostic and Statistical Manual of Mental Disorders,* third edition (*DSM-III;* American Psychiatric Association 1980) as "borderline personality disorder." It is treated even today by most practitioners with variations on psychoanalytically oriented psychotherapy.

The same process of blaming the illness as opposed to the treatment has taken place in recent years in psychopharmacology. Antidepressants were seen in the 1990s as the ultimate cure for depression. It seemed that all we needed to do to solve the problem of depression was to diagnose more people and to prescribe more antidepressants. This approach, coincidentally profitable for pharmaceutical companies as well as for incomes of psychiatric practitioners, seemed to improve the lives of many persons. However, some simply did not respond. Instead of concluding that antidepressants were perhaps not the solution for such persons (not to mention part of the problem) the profession has focused on the concept of "treatment-resistant depression." The solution: more antidepressants, combined in a different way, or perhaps electroconvulsive therapy or surgical interventions such as vagus nerve or deep brain stimulation. It may turn out that some of these treatment-resistant depressions will in fact respond to such aggressive interventions, but clearly many do not. While all illnesses possess virulent forms that are not responsive to appropriate treatments, it is medically incorrect to ignore the possibility that some, if not most, nonresponse may be due to incorrect diagnoses.

Galen once said that if his treatments failed, then the disease was incurable. This ancient error is playing out again today. The problem of treatment-resistant depression is completely analogous to the vagaries of pseudoneurotic schizophrenia and borderline personality. When a single dogma is applied to all of psychiatry, treatment-resistant syndromes will abound. It matters little whether the dogma is Freud or Effexor.

Thoughtless Psychopharmacology

The problem in the world of psychiatry today can be stated simply if indelicately: most psychopharmacologists (meaning most psychiatrists) *do not think*. They do not even think that they need to think. At least psychoanalysis was consciously a theory; and as a theory it required that its adepts study its content, which consisted of much psychology and some philosophy. Psychopharmacologists often practice with little more than a smattering of biochemical knowledge. The average psychiatrist knows little more than a well-versed layperson about neurotransmitters such as serotonin or their effects on receptors in the brain. The advanced academic may know more about second messengers and genetic or physiological effects of medications, yet most of this knowledge has little practical relevance. The basics of clinical psychopharmacology can be taught and learned in about a year of weekly classes, as I have taught for psychiatry residents and then supplemented by continuing medical education with little difficulty.

Psychopharmacology is not a complex discipline in its practical clinical aspects (though it is indeed complex with respect to science). Even so, many psychiatrists have only a moderate familiarity with this knowledge. They do not study nosology (the science of diagnosis); they do not study their conceptual assumptions in deciding to prescribe, or not to prescribe, medications; they do not think about why and whether to combine medications with psychotherapies in some cases, or not to do so in others.

Psychiatrists practice psychopharmacology as if it is simple and straightforward. No wonder psychologists and social workers and nurses think they should be given the right to prescribe. Most psychiatrists approach psychopharmacology so simply that almost anyone could do it that way.

The problem is that this simple-minded psychopharmacology is harmful. In my view (in contrast to anti-psychiatry groups like Scientology), psychopharmacology itself is not harmful; yet psychopharmacology can be, and often is, practiced in a harmful way.

Dogmatic Psychopharmacology

The reason psychopharmacology today is often harmful is because it represents a dogmatic philosophy of psychiatry. The late Paul Roazen became persona non grata in the psychoanalytic community when, in the heyday of psychoanalytic power of the late 1960s, he dared to suggest that Freud was other than the cultlike ideal he had been made out to be (Roazen 1993). Freud analyzed his own daughter; he gossiped to patients about their siblings, who were also his patients; he intervened in his disciples' love lives often to their detriment; he was cold and callous toward a brilliant student who then committed suicide (an event hushed up by Anna Freud and her coterie for fifty years; Roazen 1993). All this Roazen discovered and published, leading to Anna Freud's comment that "Everything Paul Roazen writes is a menace" (Roazen 1993). Yet Roazen was debunking Freud to save psychoanalysis, not to destroy it. No man could spend an entire career trying to understand a movement without having, at his core, sympathy for its key concepts.

When I got to know Paul Roazen decades later, he was unhappy with the evolution of psychiatry. Certainly, the excesses of psychoanalysis had ended, but they had been replaced by a psychopharmacological extremism that was equally dogmatic. "Why is everyone getting Prozac?" he would ask, implying that some would have benefited from psychotherapies instead. "Why is neurosis no longer used diagnostically?" he would ask, implying that our current nosology had lost the ability to explain many clinical syndromes. "Is lithium always effective?" he would ask, implying that it was used in cases in which patients did not have manic-depressive illness. "Is depression always a disease?" he would ask, implying that depressive syndromes were sometimes part of existence and in fact could be beneficial in some ways and, thus, that the complete eradication of all depression was not necessarily worthwhile either for individuals or for society.

What I gathered from his unease was not that psychopharmacology was inherently useless—and neither is psychoanalysis—but that its dogmatic application is fraught with harm, as was the case with psychoanalytic hegemony.

We have replaced a psychoanalytic dictator with a pharmaceutical demagogue. This has occurred despite the BPS model, which has not stopped this process, despite its frequent invocation, and never will. Much as Adolf Meyer stood by powerlessly as lobotomy swept the land, the much more benign but equally mistaken excesses of psychopharmacology are occurring without any coherent response based on the BPS model.

Has the model itself contributed to this state of affairs?

Biopsychosocial Psychopharmacology and Depression

In the compilation from Engel's disciples at the University of Rochester, only one chapter tried to apply Engel's biopsychosocial approach to psychiatric treatment, as opposed to general medicine, and it is noteworthy that the illness chosen was depression. Recall that the BPS model was mostly applied to psychosomatic syndromes: Engel himself wrote little about depression, and Roy Grinker applied the biopsychosocial model to schizophrenia; yet many clinicians today seem to see depression as a classic vehicle for the BPS approach. The author presents two versions of a case of depressive illness (deGruy 2003). The first is somewhat self-consciously backward, a "1950 version": "Vonda McGuire is 38 years old and is tired. . . . The psychiatrist confirms the diagnosis of depression and they embark on a three-year course of dynamic psychotherapy. . . . At the end of three years, Ms. McGuire is relatively free of depressive symptoms (after nearly two hundred sessions) . . . and her fatigue is improved but not eliminated. At the end of four years she notes a worsening of her fatigue and returns to her family doctor."

The "2003 version":

Vonda McGuire is 38 years old and she is tired. . . . [Her primary care physician, or PCP, diagnoses depression] and they agree to begin an SSRI antidepressant if she is not significantly better in one month. At one month . . . her physician adds sertraline . . . [The PCP meets with her and her husband who] reluctantly agrees to revise his work schedule in order to be more available to his family. She takes sertraline for one year, which causes her symptoms to remit. At the end of this time she tapers off the sertraline, experiences the first signs of her depressive symptoms returning, and resumes sertraline permanently. [The PCP then arranges family therapy to help with her husband's schedule conflicts at work and home]. . . . At the end of four years, Ms. McGuire . . . is asymptomatic. . . . Her family life is demanding but manageable. (pp. 84–95)

The author emphasizes that the key difference between the two vignettes is that in 2003 the primary care physician collaborated with the family therapist, whereas in 1950 the psychoanalytic psychiatrist tried to handle everything. "As the biopsychosocial clinician contemplates the source of this complaint, she does not strive to find the single etiologic agent. She instead considers contributions from all three domains. . . . When the complexity of the problem demands it, she collaborates with a colleague with the same biopsychosocial orientation but with deeper expertise in relationship issues. Without this collaboration, each professional ascribes primacy to her own sphere of expertise, and the interactions between the two spheres, which is where most of the explanatory power lies, is managed well by neither" (deGruy 2003). Such interdisciplinary collaboration is seen by the Rochester tradition as a hallmark of the BPS model. Again, this contrasts with recent claims by psychoanalytically oriented psychiatrists that this model justifies single clinician treatment (i.e., a psychiatrist providing both medication and psychotherapy), which is seen as more effective than split clinician treatment (a psychiatrist for medications and a psychologist or social worker for psychotherapy; Gabbard and Kay 2001). This assumption in fact conflicts with Engel's biopsychosocial tradition.

The underlying assumption of the BPS model is that multicausality is the case with mental disorders; single causes are rarely relevant. I would suggest another aspect to this case, especially as related to the decision to use sertraline. Serotonin reuptake inhibitor (SRI) antidepressants, like all medications, are not benign; they can even cause suicidality (Hammad, Laughren, and Racoosin 2006); thus, we need good reasons to use them. Symptomatic use is insufficient, especially if drugs are given indefinitely as in this case. These agents also have withdrawal syndromes; relapse to depression after stopping the SRI may not mean that the patient had a depressive illness—it could also mean that the patient became biologically dependent on the drug (Baldessarini, Ghaemi, and Viguera 2002). (This does not mean that a psychological addiction occurs; however, physical tolerance and withdrawal appears to happen.) The medical tradition dating to Hippocrates, and as interpreted in modern times by William Osler (see chapter 12), would require that we use medications primarily for diseases. What is the disease in this case? If we wish to use SRI antidepressants, the relevant disease for which they have some proof of efficacy is recurrent unipolar major depressive episodes. If a person has this condition, then the SRI should be effective, and there is little evidence that family therapy or other interventions are necessary. It is not that such psychotherapies may not be helpful; rather, they are not necessary. In contrast, antidepressants appear to be necessary. Thus, there is not equivalent multicausality: the biological component is primary in such cases. If the individual does not have the disease of recurrent unipolar depression, then there is no inherent need for sertraline (it may be useful short-term symptomatically, or perhaps not; and it is not necessary to use continuously for the long-term), and the person is likely to improve with family therapy and other nonmedication interventions, thereby sparing the risks of taking such drugs. The problem with the BPS approach is that it is overinclusive: everyone gets everything, along with all the risks and costs that come along with potentially unnecessary treatment. Prioritization of treatment methods does not happen.

To provide empirical support for the BPS model in depression, the author cites the Medical Outcomes Study of the 1980s as "the most powerful empirical demonstration in clinical medicine of the relationship between the biological, psychological, and social spheres" (deGruy 2003). The study assessed common ambulatory medical conditions, including depression, and noted their effects not just on physical symptoms but on psychological and social function. The fact that medical illnesses, some of which are almost purely biological in etiology, affect psychological states and social function is a truism; it provides no deep secret as to the nature of such mental illnesses as severe depression and schizophrenia.

The author ends his chapter dogmatically: "we can conclude that mental disorders, such as depression, are thoroughly biopsychosocial in nature" (deGruy 2003). We can?

Psychopharmacology Awry

Psychiatry, in practice, is mostly psychopharmacology. The BPS model, designed mostly to protect a space for psychotherapies, has not been able to inform the practice of psychopharmacology in any credible manner. Its effect has been, instead, to justify an eclectic liberalism in the symptomatic use of psychiatric medications. Psychiatrists have, to a large extent, given up on the medical tradition of *first* identifying diagnoses that reflect diseases and *then* providing proven treatments for those diseases. In the BPS approach, it is sufficient to provide medications for symptoms, such as antidepressants for depressive symptoms of any variety, and then to proceed to psychosocial interventions as well. This has produced an anarchic world of practice, where the Hippocratic philosophy of avoiding treatments when possible is now ignored. Medications are everywhere, for better or worse—and often for worse—partly thanks to biopsychosocial eclecticism. The result in practice has proven unsatisfactory to many, including the most important constituency: patients. As a consequence, as described in the next chapter, a reaction against contemporary psychiatry is taking place but without awareness that the BPS model itself is a large part of the problem.

CHAPTER TEN

The Vagaries of the Real World

German philosopher Georg Hegel argued that all theories, if taken logically to their full conclusion, would end in contradictions, producing the opposite of what they intended. The biopsychosocial model suffers from this Hegelian tragedy. It began as a way to avoid dogmatism, but it has ended in a new dogma; due to its broadness and vagueness, it provides no arguments against any dogma and no resistance to other forces in society that propound their particular dogmas. A case can be made that the strongest such forces in contemporary American society are the insurance and pharmaceutical industries. It is in their economic interest to propound a biologically oriented psychiatry, one in which disease labels are used widely and treated with medications (which is cheaper than psychosocial interventions for the insurance industry and a source of profits for the pharmaceutical industry). While it is not itself a cause of these forces, the biopsychosocial (BPS) model has failed to stem the devolution of psychiatry into a more and more biological field. The leaders of the profession proclaim fealty to biopsychosocial eclecticism, but the reality on the ground is biological dogmatism. Patients know this, and they are reacting.

Thus, in its role as George Engel's "design for action," the BPS model has again failed to fulfill its promise. This revival of dogmatism has occurred despite the model, which has proven powerless to resist it. The weakness of the BPS approach partly has to do with the fact that its adherents have used it in a confusing manner when thinking about its role in understanding etiology (the nature of disease) versus treatment. Engel certainly seemed to emphasize the BPS model as a way of understanding the etiology of disease, yet both he and Roy Grinker Sr. also saw it as a basic model of treating mental illness. This back and forth between seeing the BPS model as one of disease and as a guide to treatment has led to confusion in psychiatric practice, which in time has left the profession unable to adequately respond to the biologically dogmatic biases of managed care insurance companies and pharmaceutical companies, as we will see.

Treatment versus Etiology

Discussions of the BPS model frequently confuse treatment with etiology. Often it is assumed that all three components must go hand in hand: thus, genetic causes should lead to biological pathogenesis and psychopharmacological treatment, whereas environmental causes should lead to psychosocial pathogenesis and psychotherapy. The matter is much more complex. Often causes are genetic but treatments environmental (even in the most genetic conditions, such as phenylketonuria, the treatment can be environmental: diet restriction). At other times, causes are environmental but treatments biological (a person who eats only Twinkies will develop coronary artery disease, which may require surgery, rather than some kind of anti-Twinkie psychotherapy). The BPS model flounders when a one-to-one correlation between type of cause and type of treatment fails to hold. If an illness is predominantly biological and genetic in etiology and pathogenesis, psychotherapeutic treatment could still be defensible and vice versa. But then, when should we do one or the other or both? The biopsychosocial model itself provides little guidance on this question.

Combined Psychotherapy/Psychopharmacology

Frequently, clinicians advocate combination psychotherapy/psychopharmacology treatment. This result is to be expected from such a broad theory, because more specific guidance is not forthcoming. (Indeed, Engel did not emphasize the need to prove psychological treatments; he *assumed* them, and primarily psychoanalytic versions [Brown 2003].) Providing a rationale for combined treatment may be, in fact, the main reason why this theory has been so attractive (G. M. Abroms 1969). There are drawbacks to combination treatment, though. From the policy perspective, if some therapies (including medications) are sometimes not necessary, then this approach is fiscally wasteful and expensive. One might argue that the rise of managed care in the early 1990s was partly a consequence of the rampant expense of combination therapy in psychiatry in the 1980s, a time when some health insurance paid for daily psychoanalysis (as was the case in Washington, D.C., for federal employees). The psychiatric profession has not been able to counter managed care on costs (partly perhaps because the biopsychosocial model does not provide any rationale on how to limit costs).

It seems reasonable to ask of a conceptual model of psychiatry that it provide a rationale, to the public as well as the profession, for what clinicians do. If our model is not convincing to legislators and insurance agents and voters, then we will have difficulty explaining why resources should be provided for our treatments. To outsiders, in the worlds of insurance and government, the biopsychosocial model, by itself, does not provide convincing reasons why combination treatment should be funded. If research studies find such benefit, then they might be convinced. But the model itself, on its own merits, has not proved convincing. It might be suggested that the BPS approach is not meant to be a cookbook of therapeutics, which raises the question of what it is that we want from a conceptual model of psychiatry. A model should provide a rationale for the basic approaches taken to treatment, though it need not itself provide the details of such treatment.

Some might suggest that empirical studies now demonstrate the benefit of combined treatment. Discussion of this literature is usually selective. The BPS model would predict that combined treatment is the most effective treatment in general (i.e., most of the time). The available research, still limited, suggests that combined medication/psychotherapy treatment may be effective in some cases or conditions (Thase 1997) but not in others (E. Frank et al. 1990). This selective efficacy is hard to reconcile with the biopsychosocial model, which advocates using a combination of approaches for almost all problems.

Psychiatric Hubris

To some extent, the emphasis on combination therapy is also meant to be a justification of psychiatry as a guild. After all, only psychiatrists, among mental health professionals, can provide combination therapy (medications and psychotherapy), because others cannot prescribe (Gabbard and Kay 2001).

Here is another irony: the BPS model partly grew out of the battles of non-MD mental health professionals to free themselves from the yoke of playing second fiddle to psychiatrists. For all their talk of mind and psychology, the psychoanalysts in their days of power were adamant that only MDs could join their ranks, and thus power in psychiatric settings was held tightly by physicians. In their struggle for freedom, psychologists and social workers partly blamed the "medical model" of mental illness; the biopsychosocial model was, for them, a practical means of asserting their professional identities. To this day, the BPS model is almost sacrosanct in social work circles; rarely are criticisms heard of it, yet it is taught differently from how psychoanalysts teach it. In fact, the irony is that the acceptance of this approach partly grew out of the rebellion of social workers and psychologists against psychiatrists (mostly psychoanalysts), but now that same model is being used by psychiatrists (mostly psychoanalysts) to assert priority and privilege among mental health professionals.

Here's a further irony: Now nonpsychiatrist professionals, especially nurses and psychologists, have reversed course, embracing the biomedical model in their battle to gain prescribing privileges. If the biopsychosocial model is accepted, they cannot be "real" biopsychosocial practitioners unless they can prescribe. If the biopsychosocial model is rejected, then they still will be handmaidens to psychiatrists.

A cynic might be tempted to say that the models are irrelevant to the search for power, riches, and prestige.

That the BPS approach is being manipulated for the pecuniary needs of psychiatric subgroups becomes more clear when one examines the practice of Engel's medical colleagues (Epstein et al. 2003). Their discussion of "focusing the approach for clinical practice" is informative in that it gets at the critical issue of how and when to privilege one aspect of the model over another. They present a complex case of an 82-year-old woman with severe inflammatory bowel disease of uncertain pathological type. She had much conflict with her adult son, had made two suicide attempts in the previous three months, and was treated by multiple specialists. She was also an immigrant from Prague, where doctors routinely did not tell patients if they had terminal illness, and she feared that she had cancer but was not being told so. She refused to go to a nursing home but was too ill to go home; surgery could help but had some mortality risk. In this complex setting, the physician had to prioritize. First, he decided that further diagnostic workup would not provide more useful information for decision making; he then engaged the patient on her cultural fears about a more serious diagnosis and convinced her otherwise; next he arranged for family therapy for the patient and her son, followed by further discussions regarding decision making. They eventually all agreed to surgery, which led to a complicated recovery, a brief unsuccessful return home, followed by nursing home placement, and continued family therapy that proved helpful to both the patient and her son as she adjusted to life with a colostomy. The authors conclude that the BPS approach in this case required more than any single physician could provide: "expertise in gastroenterology, psychiatry, family therapy, nutrition, anthropology, and conflict resolution all seemed necessary." Thus, the BPS model does not privilege the physician per se as being more able than other providers to give biopsychosocial care; rather the role of the primary physician was to coordinate it all, and to guide along whatever aspect of care needed the most attention at any one time. In this case, cultural factors initially received separate attention, later followed by biological (surgery), and psychological (family therapy) factors.

As presented, this kind of complex case obviously calls for more than any single approach; yet, as the authors admit implicitly, some decisions still need to be made about when and where to emphasize the different factors. Not all of them can be used at any one time or all together all the time. It is precisely in this deciding between factors where the BPS model, as a result to its wish to be all-inclusive, fails.

Applying this lesson to psychiatry, it is relevant that many psychiatrists, especially psychoanalytically trained practitioners, do not have special expertise in psychopharmacology, and recently trained psychiatrists often have little expertise in psychotherapies. In contrast, clinical psychologists receive extensive training in psychotherapies, and social workers study and practice social interventions at length. It takes a great deal of effort to be a good psychopharmacologist or psychotherapist or social worker, with the highest level of expertise often gained in only one diagnostic or treatment subtype. Just as in medicine, specialization has happened in the mental health professions, although generalists also exist and have a role as well. Conceptually, it is not clear to me why combined treatment from a generalist is *always*, or even usually, better than separate treatment from highly trained persons in different specialties. BPS proponents in psychiatry who make this claim are going against the actual viewpoints of Engel, Grinker, and their students.

Postmodern Psychiatry and the Recovery Movement

Thus, the biopsychosocial model has failed to prevent economic forces that promote biological dogmatism, and attempts to use this approach to support combination treatment, and specifically to protect a role for psychotherapies, appear conceptually unsound. Indeed, the "recovery" movement and other postmodernist influenced critiques have gained force partly due to the failure of the BPS model to stem the tide of biologically oriented psychiatry.

Postmodernist interpretations of psychiatry have focused on the power structures that underlie the practice of psychiatry. The most famous of these interpretations can be found in the work of Michel Foucault (1988). Other predecessors, often grouped under the term *antipsychiatry,* include R. D. Laing (1969) and Thomas Szasz (1970). Contemporary critics, while not overtly rejecting the concept of mental illness as does Szasz, have reformulated many of the critiques of the antipsychiatry movement. Recent works in this vein have included the writings of David Healy (1998, 2006), who has argued that a "corporate psychiatry" has developed, heavily influenced by the pharmaceutical industry. Others, especially in the United Kingdom (Moncrieff 2006), argue that modern psychiatry has become a handmaiden to conservative (or "neoliberal" in the British context) political commitments. Treating the unhappiness of the masses, which derives from poverty and racism and other sociopolitical causes, as if they are biological entities, not only diverts the masses from the real causes of their discontent but enriches capitalist entities directly (i.e., the pharmaceutical and insurance companies).[1]

These approaches represent a reaction of some psychiatrists to the failures of biopsychosocial eclecticism. In distinction to this, the patient advocacy movement has begun to coalesce around the "recovery" movement, which derives from the 12-step approach to behavior (such as Alcoholics Anonymous; Davidson, Lawless, and Leary 2005). In this perspective, the goal is full recovery: a complete return to normal mental and physical states, whereby one relinquishes the role of patienthood and resumes simply being a person. The current psychiatric model of simply alleviating symptoms is not enough.[2] Recovery requires the active involvement of the person with the illness, not simply their passively receiving medical care from professionals. The recovery movement implies that the psychiatric profession has not appreciated, and thus not sufficiently abetted, the ability of persons with mental illness to get well. Though implicitly critical of mainstream psychiatry, this approach has garnered support from many community psychiatrists (Sowers 2005), as well as the leadership of the American Psychiatric Association (Sharfstein 2005). It has also appealed to many in less medically based professions, such as social work, as well as groups generally critical of psychiatry.

The recovery movement, in what could be perceived as an irony, received a stamp of approval from former president George W. Bush's New Freedom Commission on Mental Health.[3] Apparently, a libertarian philosophy of self-help, and thus less need for provision of medical care, appeals to American political conservatives. American right-wing conservatives and British left-wing critics agree on a critique of biological psychiatry; this alliance of extremes is surprising and powerful, putting biological psychiatrists on the defensive. Yet it is not unprecedented; as recent historical scholarship has shown, antipsychiatry movements have existed for at least a hundred years, beginning in Germany in the late nineteenth century (Engstrom 2004), and, at that time also, those critics came both from left-wing and right-wing political perspectives.

One might critique the recovery movement on two grounds. On one hand, its proponents often claim to support the biopsychosocial model; but if this model is part of the problem, it will not serve them well. On the other hand, the recovery concept itself has become a dogma in the hands of some of its advocates, and like any one-sided dogma, it is likely to fail if its extreme proponents deny the reality of all biologically based psychiatric disease. In that sense, the recovery dogma is perilously close to simply being another variation on antipsychiatry—a popular, perennial, and false fad.

The fact that power, economics, and politics permeate society is as old as Aristotle and as recent as Marx. These aspects of the postmodernist/semisocialist critique may be valid, though not novel. The reduction of mental illness *entirely* to social constructs, however, is another matter. Not *all* of these critics engage in this kind of postmodernist dogmatism, but many do. As Paul McHugh once wrote, it is sufficient to interview and treat a person with schizophrenia over time to realize that postmodernist dogmas are wrong (McHugh 2006). E. O. Wilson, pointing out the nihilism of postmodern extremism, commented: "Scientists, being held responsible for what they say, have not found postmodernism useful" (Dennett 1998). Postmodernist critiques likely have had both positive and negative consequences: positive in opposing the biological reductionism and capitalist ethos of much of mainstream psychiatry and negative in providing a simplistically false alternative.

Clearly, there are limitations to science, and science is influenced by sociopolitical factors; yet this does not invalidate science. Philosopher Daniel Dennett, using religion as his contrast, draws this distinction: "The irony is that these fruits of scientific reflection, showing us the ineliminable smudges of imperfection, are sometimes used by those who are suspicious of science as their grounds for denying it a privileged status in the truth-seeking department—as if the institutions and practices they see competing with it were no worse off in these regards. But where are the examples of religious orthodoxy being simply abandoned in the face of irresistible evidence? Again and again in science, yesterday's heresies have become today's new orthodoxies. No religion exhibits that pattern in its history" (Dennett 1998). There is a major danger in replacing science, properly understood in all its limitations, with any ideology—be it postmodern, postpsychiatry, antipsychiatry, recovery-oriented, libertarian, anticapitalist, or procapitalist. My own perspective is that any kind of dogmatism, or belief that one perspective has a monopoly on knowledge, is bound to fail in psychiatry, and that dogmatisms of left and right are similar. The problem is how to reject dogmatism while also avoiding the pitfall of eclecticism.

Part of the Solution or Part of the Problem?

In contrast to my diagnosis of the BPS model as part of the problem, many still see it as the solution to current problems in the field. For instance, one proponent argues that the excessive influence of the pharmaceutical industry is due to the biomedical model: "A clinical medicine devoid of its psychosocial dimension and therefore extremely liable to corporate influences . . . [is] a dehumanized, technological medicine, loaded with conflict of interest and with marketing strategies" (Fava 2006). The same claim is made, without much elaboration, by other critics of the pharmaceutical industry in primary care medicine (Abramson 2008).

What these critics fail to explain, especially in psychiatry, is how the BPS model can be proposed as a solution when, for the past two decades, these problems have arisen while it has been universally acclaimed in mainstream American psychiatry. This would be like Mikhail Gorbachev blaming the poor economic state of the former Soviet Union on lack of adherence to communist doctrine. The claim that the BPS model was not sufficiently used in general medicine might be more convincing, but, in psychiatry, it has had more or less free play for the past few decades. Its failures are only its own.

Part III / What Next?

CHAPTER ELEVEN

The Limits of Evidence-Based Medicine

Some psychiatrists seem more inclined to reinterpret the biopsychosocial model, rather than to give it up, along something like the following lines: "The BPS model has not lived up to its expectations, it is true," they might say. "But it really should not be placed at such high expectations. We view the model as a general framework for our field. It reminds us to pay attention to all three components of human behavior. We then use the principles of evidence based medicine to evaluate those components."

This view has some superficial appeal. It shifts the emphasis from a general model (the biopsychosocial approach) to a general method (evidence-based medicine [EBM]). An added appeal is that EBM was developed in general medicine, and thus, like the BPS model, it would connect psychiatry to that field.

The problem is that this approach to EBM is nothing but the biological dogma dressed up in new clothes, another example of how the eclecticism of the BPS model can be used to cloak underlying dogmatism.

Evidence-Based Medicine and the Loss of the Subjective

EBM has become perhaps the most popular potential replacement for the biopsychosocial approach. If this replacement was to be complete, especially in any simplistic way, we would be taking a step backward, moving from eclecticism to another variety of dogmatism.

EBM in particular can be abused because of its predilection for privileging objective data, leading to an overemphasis on research and attention to those areas of psychiatry where objective data are more easily attained, such as biological and psychopharmacological fields. In recent years, about 90 percent of published articles in psychiatric journals about bipolar disorder, for instance, have been biological or psychopharmacological in content. Only about 10 percent involved psychotherapies, psychosocial aspects, psychopathology, or nosology (Soldani, Ghaemi, and Baldessarini 2005). This is a reflection of the inherent bias of the objective-empirical method (with EBM as a prime example) toward nonsubjective aspects of psychiatry.

One psychiatric leader (van Praag 1980) has asked the following question: what is psychiatry without subjectivity? For it is precisely the subjective components of mental illness that identify psychiatry as a profession, as opposed to neurology or medicine. If mental illness were to be purely reduced to objective signs and symptoms or neuroscience-based correlates, we would observe the same process as happened with the transformation of chronic psychosis into neurosyphilis or the same process as happened with the transformation of senile psychosis into Alzheimer's dementia with the definition of its underlying neuropathology. In those cases— where psychological syndromes are directly due to biological abnormalities of the brain, and nothing else—indeed the work of the psychiatrist is the same as the work of any physician, and no distinction between psychiatry and neurology, between mental illness and brain disease, can be drawn.

More than a century of careful biological research has demonstrated that the same cannot be said for a handful of psychotic and affective conditions that we call schizophrenia and manic-depressive illness. While these conditions clearly have biological preconditions, they are not reducible to their biological causes and thus have important environmental and psychosocial components, both in their genesis and to some extent in their treatment. These are biologically based conditions, but, I am emphasizing that they cannot be *reduced* to biological brain diseases. Part of this inability to reduce these illnesses to objective aspects of disease has to do with the subjective experience of these conditions. People have unique and important experiences in the course of have a psychotic episode or being manic or depressed; recognition and understanding of these subjective experiences is an important part of being able to make these diagnoses. Even though treatment is largely pharmacological, subjective aspects of allying with these individuals and helping them as they go through the process of treatment and recovery is key to the success of pharmacological treatment. While applauding the need for EBM viewed as scientific medicine—the application of our most advanced statistical and epidemiological methods to medicine—we cannot pretend that changing the name of objective empirical (scientific) medicine makes it anything more than the single method (albeit a powerful one) that it is.

What Is Evidence?

Perhaps the most critical issue within the concept of EBM is to appropriately understand the notion of "evidence." David Sackett, a founder of EBM, initially wanted to call it "scientific-based medicine" but settled on the word "evidence" (Sackett et al. 2000). Yet, as noted above, objective evidence is much easier to obtain than is subjective evidence. And such objective evidence is often greater in quantity if it results from research funds provided by groups that have an interest in producing such evidence. The reality is that the pharmaceutical industry provides the research funds for almost all treatment research that happens in clinical psychopharmacology. The "evidence" available to be assessed is usually greater for agents that are marketed by those companies than other agents, such as generic drugs, which are not marketed and thus not targeted for research funding. Pharmaceutical companies do not generally provide funding for psychotherapies or psychosocial treatments, and, because those treatments have important subjective components, studies of psychotherapies and psychosocial interventions are generally more complex and more expensive than psychopharmacology studies. The result is that there is much more "evidence" for psychopharmacological treatments, especially of drugs marketed currently by pharmaceutical companies, compared with either older drugs or with psychotherapies or psychosocial interventions. Still, this greater evidence is not a reflection of proven superiority but rather an absence of evidence for the older drugs or the psychosocial interventions.

Often the concept of EBM is misunderstood, or consciously abused by the pharmaceutical industry, to make this absence of evidence appear to be proof of superiority. For instance, the acclaimed Cochrane Collaboration meta-analyses in the United Kingdom, which are heavily funded by the U.K. National Health Service, privilege new drugs over older drugs and over psychotherapies for the above reasons. They simply review the available data, and these data are presented as the best evidence, which implies that other agents or treatments not included have less evidence or are proven less valid. In fact, those meta-analyses run the risk of misconstruing the economic and political forces driving research funding as a basis for claiming more or less of an evidence base for certain treatments. Some call this "evidence-biased medicine" (Evans 1995).

Ivory-Tower Evidence-Based Medicine

In the scientific world of academia, one frequently encounters an ivory-tower EBM—the belief that evidence-based medicine simply means the presence of the most rigorous kind of scientific research: double-blind, placebo-controlled studies. This interpretation is both incorrect and harmful, yet it is prevalent. Here we see another problem with EBM: Like the BPS model, it has become a catchphrase that many use for their own purposes. For academic scientists, it can be convenient to simply ignore all kinds of evidence if it does not meet that double-blind, placebo-controlled standard; this is much easier than the hard scientific work of actually comparing different levels of evidence.

This ivory-tower EBM is incorrect because the central insight of evidence-based medicine is the need to know and apply the highest level of *available* evidence to clinical practice, not the application of only the highest level of *possible* evidence. Ivory-tower EBM is harmful because many academics use this misinterpretation to privilege the studies that they find most acceptable for the reasons given above. Double-blind, placebo-controlled studies are expensive and thus more likely to happen where funding sources, such as with the pharmaceutical industry, exist. Drugs are much more easily studied in such paradigms than psychotherapies. Also, such research designs are not feasible for some important questions: based on this kind of ivory-tower EBM, we could never *prove* that cigarette smoking causes lung cancer, just as we cannot prove that lithium prevents suicide. Ivory-tower EBM dogmatism would thus conclude that we neither have enough evidence to regulate and minimize cigarette smoking nor enough to recommend lithium for suicide prevention (Soldani, Ghaemi, and Baldessarini 2005).

Eclecticism has many faults, but it has fewer than any type of dogma.

Method-Based Psychiatry

A better alternative would be what I will call "method-based psychiatry," in contrast to evidence-based medicine. This is the same notion that I describe elsewhere as "pluralism" in contrast to BPS eclecticism (see chapter 16 and glossary). Method-based psychiatry would take the view that what matters are our methods not our theories. In fact, our methods determine our theories and our facts; as Karl Jaspers put it, between fact and method no sharp line can be drawn. The key issue, then, is to know when to use the appropriate method. For some conditions or circumstances, an objective-descriptive biological method is appropriate; in other conditions or circumstances, a psychological method of a certain kind (such as existential phenomenology) may be more appropriate. We need to know which method should be used where, based on empirical scientific evidence as much as possible (in agreement with EBM) but also based on conceptual rationales. The contrast with current thinking is that EBM is a single method, the objective-descriptive empirical approach, and thus does not apply for all conditions or circumstances. If we reject dogmatism, then we have to reject EBM as a solution for our ills. We do not then have to revert to BPS eclecticism. We have a noneclectic, nondogmatic alternative: a method-based psychiatry (see chapter 16).

To summarize: the concept of evidence-based medicine is not fundamentally flawed, but it tends to be misunderstood by clinicians and researchers alike. Its misuse by those with pecuniary interests needs to be acknowledged and combated. Despite its strengths, its limitations are such that, either added to or in place of the BPS model, it is far from a general conceptual model for psychiatry.

CHAPTER TWELVE

Osler's Ghost

A specter hovers over this debate, the spirit of the person with arguably the greatest influence on medical education in the past century, a man widely viewed as the founder of modern scientific medicine: William Osler. Osler's ghost reminds us that the biopsychosocial (BPS) approach is not the only alternative to a dehumanized biomedical model. The biomedical model that George Engel set himself against was something of a straw man: Engel kept emphasizing that patients were tired of medicine being *only* technological, uninterested in human beings, dehumanized. In examining the attraction of his students to the BPS model (chapter 5), we saw that they were largely drawn to it as a humanistic alternative to the biomedical model. Engel himself resisted this line of reasoning. He insisted that the BPS model was not simply a humanistic philosophy but rather *more* scientific than the biomedical model—an extension of scientific methods from biology into the psychosocial worlds as well. We also saw in chapter 2 how Ludwig von Bertalanffy, the leading exponent of general systems theory (GST, often seen as the philosophical basis for the BPS model), ridiculed humanistic approaches to psychology as variations on countercultural hippiedom.

The pretenses of Engel and von Bertalanffy's are all fluff. Engel's view of the science of psychology involved psychoanalytic theories that can hardly be called scientific by most definitions of that term. GST also has not panned out as the scientific basis of modern biology. As scientific programs, Engel's BPS and von Bertalanffy's GST have failed. If instead one supports the BPS model on humanistic grounds, not only is that view explicitly opposed to Engel's perspective but also one has to explain how it improves on another alternative: the biomedical model with humanism added to it—the ghost of William Osler.

William Osler the Man

The mention of William Osler in medical circles these days tends to produce two mental associations: medical humanism and the importance of clinical examination (that is, bedside teaching and careful observation of clinical cases; Osler 1948). Osler is justifiably regarded as a modern Hippocrates, if we see a major feature of the Hippocratic worldview as the notion that we should rely on observation of cases, rather than theory, as the basis for medical judgment. Like Hippocrates, Osler emphasized a conservative approach to practice, erring on the side of nontreatment in doubtful situations so as to avoid inflicting unnecessary harm (Bliss 1999; McHugh 1987).

Ironically, given his later fame as a medical humanist, what was unique about Osler in his early career was that he was widely seen as a leader in the introduction of scientific methods into modern medicine. In the late nineteenth century, clinical use of the microscope was new, as was pathological autopsy. These two factors revolutionized medicine. By opening the body after death and examining the tissue microscopically, the pathologist could actually *see* the disease. He could then give a verdict, like an all-knowing deity: the clinician's diagnosis before death was either right or wrong. This is the famous "clinicopathological" method in medicine, and Osler, perhaps more than anyone, implemented it (Bliss 1999).

The clinicopathological method was revolutionary partly because it did away with medical eclecticism: I could not have my diagnosis and theory of disease, and you your diagnosis and theory of disease—the pathologist would tell us who was right and who was wrong. There was a truth to the matter, and no one could deny the verdict of the microscope.

Osler was both pathologist and clinician. He spent countless hours dissecting bodies and showing students the inner workings of pathological study;[1] yet he spent even more hours at the bedside observing signs and symptoms, obtaining history, and making diagnostic judgments. Osler's scientific genius was that he was a stellar clinical diagnostician and a superb pathologist: so he could observe patients clinically for extended periods of time, and after they died, he himself would look inside those patients' bodies and determine if he had been right or wrong. If wrong, Osler would adjust his clinical approach until he became more and more accurate in his diagnosis, as confirmed at autopsy (Bliss 1999).

Osler then took this clinical experience to students, popularizing bedside teaching. In his famed medical "rounds," he would go from patient to patient followed by a horde of students observing his diagnostic approach. Osler insisted that clinical skill needed to be learned in real life in the hospitals, not books (Osler 1948).

These then made Osler justly famous: the introduction of the clinicopathological method and the emphasis of bedside clinical teaching. Add his sparkling personality, and Osler was a man bound for greatness—he was called to be the first chair of medicine at the newly formed Johns Hopkins Hospital in 1895, and soon thereafter he wrote a classic textbook of medicine that would be used extensively for half a century.

Osler's Reductionism

Some have criticized Osler, though, for being *too* reductionist. This hard-core Osler is insufficiently appreciated, in fact, by many contemporary physicians, for whom Osler seems like a romantic relic. Yet the critique is made by those who are aware of how Osler was indeed a biologically oriented revolutionary come to clean up an eclectic medicine. Here is the view of a historian of medicine who sympathizes with Engel: "The 'Osler line' moved in a reductionist, biological direction. Medicine was an experimental science and the human organism—as Abraham Flexner put it in his famous Flexner Report of 1910—was not essentially different from a *frog*" (italics in original; Brown 2000). Osler's successor as chair of internal medicine at Johns Hopkins, Lewellys F. Barker, was more psychologically inclined: "When Barker took over clinical and teaching responsibilities from Osler, he found one major area of deficiency. This is how he remembered the situation in his autobiography: 'Admirable as Dr. Osler's organization and conduct of the clinic had been, there was one field that had been inadequately cultivated, namely, that of the functional nervous disorders. . . . When patients manifested symptoms of these disorders they were often rather lightly referred to as being 'neurotics' and received too little attention from either staff or students. . . . Dr. Osler had been trained in the pathological-anatomical school, and he was more particularly interested in organic rather than in functional disorders of the nervous system'" (Brown 2000).

Indeed, if one peruses Osler's textbook of medicine, on the one hand, one can note that his section on psychiatric conditions is brief and reserved, with discussions of "neurasthenia" and hysteria, and polite skepticism about psychoanalytic theory. On the other hand, Osler was friendly with Silas Weir and a proponent of diagnosing and treating neurasthenia with Weir's "rest cure." So it is not that Osler was uninterested in neuroses; rather, he preferred to separate them off for supportive management and then to focus on those organic conditions for which cures were available. Osler even once corresponded with Freud about sending a patient for consultation, after his arrival in England; this brief interaction did not appear to greatly impress either genius (Bliss 1999).

Osler was reductionistic, when it came to biology, but he supplemented this biological reductionism with a medical humanism that complemented it. In contrast, the nonreductionistic speculations of psychoanalytic theory—whether by Freud or Barker or Engel—were nonscientific, and, ultimately, nonhumanistic. Osler's medical humanism, which supplemented his biological reductionism, is the important second half of the picture.

Osler's Medical Humanism

After achieving this scientific fame, Osler led a second revolution in modern medicine: medical humanism. The emphasis on pathology that Osler inculcated always raised the danger of viewing the patient as a conglomeration of organs and nothing more. Soon, the rise of laboratory tests further attracted many students to the notion that medical practice could consist of tests and autopsy. Against this trend, Osler emphasized the need to stick to the clinical examination and history: pathology and laboratory tests, though helpful, served mainly to improve, not to replace, clinical skills at the bedside. In his later career, Osler was increasingly out of touch with new scientific methods, particularly laboratory-based research; instead, moving to Oxford to be Regius Professor of Medicine in 1906, Osler spent the next thirteen years of his life advocating a humanistic approach to medical practice (Bliss 1999). He reminded his students that they treated the person, not the disease. In addition to laboratory tests and pathological autopsy, they needed to pay close attention to the clinical history and symptoms of the living patient. Even more, they needed to pay attention to the wishes, beliefs, and fears of the person who had the disease. Osler resuscitated the Hippocratic view that medicine consisted of three factors: the patient, the disease, and the doctor. Medicine was not just about the disease—it involved the person as well (Shorter 2005).

Osler was overtly humanistic: he had no pretensions of trying to apply scientific methods to our understanding of persons. His sources were literary, perhaps partly influenced by his Anglophilia: much of Shakespeare, British Orientalist Richard Burton, Scottish essayist Thomas Carlyle, and more than a touch of the ancients (Osler 1948). Osler divided medical knowledge, then, into two parts: scientific and humanistic.

The scientific part related to diseases and was based on the sciences of pathology, laboratory medicine, and clinical observation. The humanistic part related to understanding the persons who had diseases and was based on literary wisdom and worldly experience with the feelings and wishes of human beings.

In short, Osler added literary humanism to the medical model: Osler's medical model was science plus humanism. In modern terms, Osler, like Engel, reacted to and opposed a dehumanized interpretation of the biomedical model; but instead of seeking to create a new medical model, as did Engel, Osler revised the medical model by adding a humanistic element.

Engel versus Osler

In a tribute published in 2001 shortly after Engel's death, his son Peter Engel, MD, emphasized the idea of relationships and listening to the person as key to the BPS model (P. A. Engel 2001). In this tribute, he cited the following sections of a paper by his father titled, "How Much Longer Must Medicine's Science Be Bound by a Seventeenth Century Worldview?" (G. L. Engel 1992):

> To appreciate relationship and dialogue as requirements for scientific study in the clinical setting highlights the natural confluence of the human and the scientific in the clinical encounter itself. It is not just that science is a human activity, it is also that the interpersonal engagement required in the clinical realm rests on complementary and basic human needs, *especially the need to know and understand and the need to feel known and understood* [italics in original]. . . . The need to know and to understand achieves its most advanced development in the disciplined curiosity that characterizes scientific thinking. The need to feel known and understood manifests itself in the continuity of human relationships and in the social complementarity between perceived helplessness and the urge to help. Herein then converge the scientific and the caring (Samaritan, pastoral) roles of the physician.

Peter Engel then states: "This is the core of the biopsychosocial model" (P. A. Engel 2001). If this is the core of the BPS model, it was just as well, if not better, explained and taught by Osler in the nineteenth century. Certainly Engel's take on the importance of attending to the psychological needs of the individual seeking treatment was informed and influenced by psychoanalytic ideas, whereas Osler obviously was not. But, over time, as BPS proponents diminished the specific psychoanalytic concepts that applied to Engel's work, their view of the BPS model came more and more to resemble Osler's medical humanism.

With this background, it can be seen that there are aspects to what Engel did that are not new and certain aspects that are more original. The part that is not new, as emphasized by medical historian Edward Shorter, has to do with medical humanism (Shorter 2005). Much of what Engel argued vis-à-vis the doctor-patient relationship and the focus on the person as opposed to the disease had been described well by Adolf Meyer, and perhaps more importantly by Osler.[2] Without ever apparently citing Osler once, Engel was making essentially the same point when he kept emphasizing the significance of relating to the patient as a person.

Engel's Antihumanism Revisited

Notwithstanding the humanistic connotations often attributed to the biopsychosocial approach, as mentioned in chapter 8, Engel clearly had no patience for humanism separated from science: He wanted to show the BPS model to be a hardheaded scientific theory that incorporates psychology and sociology, not simply as a humanistic art. He made this point most clearly in a late paper, published in 1992, in which he begins to sound exasperated that the BPS model has not been adequately accepted (G. L. Engel 1992): "The fundamental issue is whether physicians can in their study and care of patients be scientists and work scientifically in the human domain. Or is medicine's human domain beyond the reach of science and the scientific method, an art, as the biomedical model in effect requires? The fundamental distinction . . . is not between 'science' and 'art' but between thinking and proceeding scientifically and not so thinking and proceeding."

Engel did not claim that the biomedical model had no utility; only that its utility needed to be limited to its sphere of relevance: "Like its 17th century counterpart in classical physics, the biomedical model represents a limiting case the utility of which is in now way diminished as long as its use is restricted to the phenomena for which it was designed. The biomedical model needs no defense, neither with respect to its past accomplishments nor to its future utility, as long as that rule is applied. But to do otherwise is to be *unscientific;* to advocate doing otherwise is to promote dogma and become *antiscientific*" (G. L. Engel 1992).

Being empathic was not enough for Engel; he wanted to invent a new scientific paradigm.

Engel insisted on including the human components of medicine consciously within the realm of science. For instance, he cites a definition of science from another physician as follows: "Science represents man's most persistent effort to extend and organize knowledge by reasoned efforts that ultimately depend on evidence that can be consensually validated" (G. L. Engel 1992).[3] This is one definition of science, but work in the history and philosophy of science suggests that there is no single definition of science, nor a single scientific method. This definition, for instance, does not specify important aspects of scientific work such as hypothesis, observation, and experiment; nor does it ask questions about induction, causality, or deductive inference. Engel's view, though not plainly positivistic, is not particularly nuanced either. Engel used Thomas Kuhn's concept of paradigms of science to claim that outgrown paradigms become dogmas and that most physicians lived in a seventeenth-century paradigm of science derived from Newton and Descartes, one that was rigid and linear and simplistic. Engel thought his approach was consistent with the twentieth-century paradigm of quantum physics, citing Heisenberg on the inherent uncertainties of knowledge. Uncertainties in psychosocial knowledge are not unscientific from a twentieth-century perspective of science. There is reason to agree with Engel on this notion that science is not simplistic, positivistic, and as untroubled by theory, hypothesis, and uncertainty as many assume; yet it seems forced to conclude that *therefore* the biopsychosocial model is valid. Why could one not still accept the biomedical approach, leavened with knowledge from psychology and sociology and other fields, including literature and the arts, as needed? Why does Engel's specific biopsychosocial model, with its commitments to general systems theory, follow? Engel contrasts the "relational mode" to the "observational mode" claiming that the dialogue of the clinical encounter is basic to the scientific enterprise. Biomedicine rejects dialogue and pretends to an objectivity it does not possess. Engel provided an example when physicians saw a patient with hemoptysis and reported an unrevealing initial history and physical examination. After a series of tests were negative, further BPS history was obtained and it was found that the patient had ingested "a bottle of Bucca" the previous night (G. L. Engel 1992). Yet Osler too was a master of observation and emphasized taking a person's clinical history above all else. He emphasized that patients "need to be known and understood" (Osler 1948), and he too probably would have discovered the bottle of Bucca.

Another example from Engel involved a patient he interviewed in grand rounds in front of many observers. The man was initially hostile and cold, as is often the case in such circumstances. After Engel approached him empathically, the patient cried at one point and the interview led to more valid information than if the he had simply been coldly questioned. Yet it is not clear to me how this example specifically supports Engel's biopsychosocial as opposed to Osler's empathic approach or existential methods in psychiatry (Ghaemi 2003; see also chapters 12 and 15 of this volume).

The Dehumanizing Effect of the Biopsychosocial Model

One might accuse Engel of a deep mistake here: he seemed to take humanism for granted. He seemed to think that if we accept the BPS model, then all the benefits of humanism would naturally follow, and we would be more scientific to boot. Yet one might claim the opposite: in at least some hands, it appears that the BPS model *is not even humanistic,* much less scientific. Can one practice the BPS model in a dehumanized, cold, and unfeeling way?

Discussing criticisms of the medical model—which come often from psychologists, social workers, and sociologists—a philosopher concluded that they mainly involved anger about a dehumanized and disrespectful approach to people with mental illness, especially in mental asylum settings (Macklin 1973). That author concluded that the problem did not seem to lie in an essential aspect of the medical model itself but rather in its application in our society. (Where does the medical model say that you should be rude and mean to your patients?) Here is the crux: advocates of the BPS model assume that by including psychosocial aspects of illness, we will become more sensitive and humane practitioners. This need not be the case.

Here are two real historical examples. In the 1960s, a predominant theory among American psychoanalysts was that much of the etiology of schizophrenia was due to harmful emotional experiences in early childhood with one's primary caretakers, which they dubbed the schizophrenogenic mother. For decades, prominent psychiatrists believed deeply, and told the public, that the mothers were to blame.

In contrast, in the 1970s and later, evidence began to accumulate that indeed there is a genetic susceptibility to schizophrenia and that biological alterations (both in anatomy and biochemistry) appear to exist in brains of persons with schizophrenia. Twin studies suggested that family environment was irrelevant to the risk to developing the condition, no psychosocial traumas could be identified as statistically related to it, and psychoanalytically oriented treatments were proven less effective.

The psychoanalysts were proven wrong. In the meantime, biologically oriented psychiatrists began to help families realize that genes and the brain were more important; those families then organized groups (like the National Alliance for the Mentally Ill), which have since had major influence in reducing stigma of mental illness in the United States.

Who was more humane—the biological psychiatrists who have reduced stigma (and been proven more correct by scientific research) or the psychoanalysts with their false theories of blame?

Here we see where a psychologically oriented approach was less humane than a biological one.

Another historical example: Philippe Pinel (who rose to influence with the French Revolution) is famous for being the founder of moral therapy in medicine; many do not appreciate that he implemented his humanistic views based on the materialism of the Enlightenment (Goldstein, Deysack, and Kleinknecht 1973). He viewed mental illness as due to abnormalities of the body and brain, not due to spiritual failings, as was the belief before his time. His humanism grew out of his materialism: again the biomedical model led to more, not less, humanism in psychiatry.

The lessons of Walter Freeman and Henry Cotton (chapter 1) also show that biological psychiatry can be dehumanizing, but the biomedical model is not inherently associated with a dehumanized approach to persons; in fact, it has been often progressive, and, in contrast, psychological or nonmedical models can be dehumanizing. The fault is not in the medical model, but rather partly in whether we use such models dogmatically and partly whether we are sensitive to those aspects of human beings that lie outside of our scientific models altogether.

Being Ill versus Having an Illness

How can Engel's BPS model encourage an antihumanistic approach to mental illness? Engel emphasizes that it is wrong to view illnesses as things that people have; rather, we must see illnesses in relation to the person—the personality as a whole. Hence, in Engel's view, one is not a person who *has* an illness—one *is* the illness. This is heard in the traditional way that medical professionals might describe an illness: "the patient *is* diabetic," we might say, instead of "the person *has* diabetes." In medical illnesses, the linguistic difference may not carry much punch, but in mental illnesses it does.

When we say, "You *are* schizophrenic," we are sending a different message from when we say, "You *have* schizophrenia"; we are sending a message that currently holds a stigma in our society. You are your illness; you are psychotic, through and through, you, poor you (Havens 1984, 1985a). What a different message from saying that you are a normal human being, just like me and everybody else, and you happen to have this disease, a disease that has happened to you, is part of you, but also is not part of you, a disease that does not constitute who you are as a human being (see chapter 17). There is more stigma with Engel's perspective; the holistic view is more blaming than the narrow biological view.

Though Engel claimed to be seeking to fight this dehumanizing approach, it seems to follow that his emphasis on *not* viewing illnesses as separate from the persons who have them would simply worsen these stigmatizing habits. Given his emphasis on science, it would seem that the biomedical approach seems more scientific, more tied to the facts, and *less prone* to judge the person who has the disease.

Here is an irony for Engel: he thinks that the biomedical approach (isolating etiologies and pathologies of disease) is often wrong scientifically (at least in chronic medical diseases) and harmful ethically; yet that approach often is right scientifically (even for chronic medical diseases) and helpful ethically (especially with stigmatized mental illnesses). In contrast, Engel assumes that the BPS model will result in more humanistic medical practice, whereas in fact it can be, and has been, used in a dehumanizing manner.

Psychoanalysis in Disguise

Some might argue that the dehumanizing uses of the BPS approach are derived from a psychoanalytic orientation, common in the 1970s and influential for Engel but less common now. The BPS model, on this view, can be modernized.

If contemporary books on psychiatric education are relevant, the BPS model is still not presented much differently from the way it was in the 1970s. For instance, in 2006, two psychiatry residency directors published a book titled *The Biopsychosocial Formulation Manual: A Guide for Mental Health Professionals* (Campbell and Rohrbaugh 2006). The 158 pages of text break down as follows: after an initial overview section, the text provides seven pages for the "biological formulation," thirty-two pages for the "psychological formulation" (divided into seventeen pages for psychoanalytic concepts, seven pages for cognitive behavioral views, and eight pages for general comments), and seven pages for the "social formulation." In other words, most of the emphasis is placed on psychological and, specifically, psychoanalytic views: one can even quantify it—contemporary supporters of the BPS model emphasize psychoanalytic approaches over two times more often than they do biological or social approaches.

One can examine the matter qualitatively as well. The short biological section of the book describes a few mnemonics for identifying clinical syndromes of depression and mania and then identifies three "biological predispositions": genetics, physical conditions, and medications/substances—that is it. The authors have little to say about the relevance of these biological components; in one paragraph they say about genetics that one should "address" (how?) the presence of mental disorders in family members, that physical conditions like "medical illnesses, neurological disorders and nonpathological states such as pregnancy" should be examined to determine whether they contribute to the mental disorder, and that substances, including over-the-counter medications, should not be overlooked. This is it for the biological component of psychiatry.

Turning to the psychological component of the BPS model, "the four components of the psychological formulation" are identified as "predisposing factors: identification of a psychological theme," "current precipitants: identification of psychosocial stressors," "psychic consequences of current psychosocial stressors: strong emotions and changes in cognition," and "dealing with stress: adaptive and maladaptive coping mechanisms." For the first section on the identification of a psychological theme, they identify "three common psychological themes": "Can I trust others to provide emotional and physical support to me? Can I remain in control of myself and control my environment? Can I maintain a healthy sense of self-esteem?" And they identify "three types of patient data that are pertinent to developing a psychological theme": "disruptions in psychological development . . . recurrent difficulties in relationships [and] revelatory statements and behavior." After a good deal of discussion about the other three components of the psychological formulation, they commence a totally new section entitled "Psychodynamic Perspective," in which the authors describe "Freud's major developmental themes": difficulties with trust or having to depend on others, difficulties with control, difficulties with self-esteem, and difficulties with triadic relationships (romantic relationships that frequently include a third person). They go on to incorporate ideas derived from Erik Erikson to identify "the four major developmental themes," which are dependency/trust, control, self-esteem, and difficulties with intimate relationships. Each of these is discussed in detail; for instance, for self-esteem, the authors write: "Not having internalized a sense of self-esteem, these people have a tendency to appear grandiose, 'narcissistic,' cold, or 'prickly.' They are outspoken, provocative, and seek positions of power and have little internal sense of themselves as worthy individuals. Difficulties in this phase may result in the development of narcissistic personality" (Campbell and Rohrbaugh 2006).

They then discuss "the psychodynamic database," which consists of an incredible level of detail: "disruptions in psychological development, recurrent difficulties in relationships, revelatory statements and behavior, current precipitants/psychosocial stressors, psychic consequences, coping mechanisms, [and] defense mechanisms." Having introduced the last concept, they now go on to provide descriptions of all the defense mechanisms, namely acting out, denial, dissociation, introjection, omnipotent control, primitive idealization (and devaluation), projection, projective identification, splitting, altruism, anticipation, blocking, controlling, displacement, externalization, humor, hypochondriasis, identification, identification with the aggressor, intellectualization, isolation of affect, passive-aggressive behavior, rationalization, reaction formation, regression, repression, sublimation, somatization, and suppression. Finally, they describe "common clinical presentations and their corresponding defense mechanisms": "antisocial personality traits—omnipotent control," "borderline personality traits—splitting, projective identification," "depression—introjection, irritability—displacement, impulsive behavior—acting out, narcissistic personality traits—primitive idealization and devaluation, paranoia—projection, and unexplained physical symptoms—somatization" (Campbell and Rohrbaugh 2006).

At last, the psychological section turns to a nonpsychoanalytic view, briefly describing the "cognitive perspective" as involving three components: "automatic dysfunctional thoughts, negative core beliefs, and cognitive distortions (errors of logic)." These are described in similar detail as the defense mechanism section. "Three components of a behavioral formulation" are also added consisting of the following questions: "Is there behavioral reinforcement of a maladaptive behavior? Is there something that extinguishes a desired behavior? Is there a paired association between a behavior and an environmental cue that initiates the behavior?"

The social formulation is then described as ten categories in a social database: family, friends/significant others, social environment, education, work, housing, income, access to health care services, legal problems/crime, and other. Each is described in a sentence. More detail is provided for "categories for the cultural and spiritual assessment" (Campbell and Rohrbaugh 2006).

It is difficult to read this supposedly definitive (according to the publisher) modern presentation of the BPS model in psychiatry without concluding that the *P* is highly privileged and that the *B* and the *S* parts of the formulation barely register and then do so blandly. Not only that: clearly the *P* stands much more for psychoanalytic ideas than anything else. This is not a BPS model, but an attempt to sneak psychoanalysis in through the back door (Shorter 2005).

Of course, the proponents of the biopsychosocial model might claim otherwise; they might claim that biological approaches are so predominant now that advocates of the biopsychosocial approach need to emphasize psychosocial components to compensate. But, as the above book demonstrates, and as I am sure social workers who might be reading these lines would wonder, one question is why they emphasize psychology over social components? And within psychology, why is psychoanalysis so distinctly emphasized over other views? Obviously, space constraints exist within any handbook, but the way one uses the space allowed is informative.

It is hard to avoid the conclusion that the BPS model, in psychiatry at least, remains a mechanism for proponents of psychoanalytic ideas to justify that approach. It is not, in fact, a larger critique of the nature of medicine (as Engel intended), nor a self-consciously critical approach to all dogmatism (as Grinker intended), nor an attempt to emphasize the social and public health aspects of illness (as it is used in social work and epidemiology).

The biopsychosocial model is, at least in psychiatry, psychoanalysis in disguise.

The Art of Medicine

After all his attacks on the biomedical model as dehumanized, it seems not entirely illegitimate to turn Engel's attacks back on the BPS model and see it as a Trojan horse for psychoanalytic dogma. The art of medical humanism, which Engel dismissed, seems much more complex and valuable than he perhaps realized. This brings us back to William Osler.

There are those who mistakenly claim Osler would have been in support of the BPS approach to medicine (Abramson 2008). This is simply historically wrong, as should now be clear, because nothing could be further from Engel's view. Osler was not, as some BPS advocates assume, simply a fuzzy-headed advocate of treating the patient as a person. Rather, he came to the fore among his colleagues for his hardheaded scientific approach to medicine; and he emphasized the need for clinical medicine to be supplemented by pathological findings, laboratory tests of blood and urine, and new methods like x-rays. Osler was all for technology, though it is also true that he emphasized the need for maintaining humane contact with the person inside the patient. Osler was also committed to seeing medicine as consisting of two separate but complementary aspects—a science and an art. Engel, in contrast, clearly opposed this view; he saw himself as a scientist and nothing more.

Engel offered two alternatives—the "biomedical model" in its most extreme form (dehumanized, cold, and technological), or the BPS model. Osler offered another choice: he similarly rejected a cold inhumane approach to medicine, but he offered the biomedical model *plus the art of medicine* as an alternative. Engel rejected this because he thought that an approach to the humanistic aspect of medicine that relies on art and literature is inferior to a scientific approach that incorporates psychology, and sociology, public health, and other disciplines. This is the real intellectual choice: Osler's medicine or Engel's medicine? In practice, the question also is, given the previous influence of Osler's view: Is there anything to Engel's BPS model that takes us further than our traditional biological approach to medicine leavened by an Oslerian appreciation of the humanities?

Criticisms of Osler

I can imagine that some of my more no-nonsense readers—medical students and doctors in particular—will find this insufficient: What are we saying? Are we just going to go back to the genteel nineteenth century, reciting poetry and worshipping Shakespeare? How is this going to help patients?

Yet those readers who might have so loved literature that they obtained degrees in those forgotten disciplines of the humanities—literature, history, the arts, writing—will sense that this question is about as meaningful as saying, "Don't you know, we have no need for water! We have H_2O!"

Nor is William Osler without his critics. My goal in invoking his ideas is not to borrow the cloak of his reputation. Too often this is the case among doctors. Doctors who hate the pharmaceutical industry cite Osler; those who support that industry cite him too. Those who opposed evidence-based medicine cite him, as do its supporters. Osler—like Freud, Marx, Heidegger, Hegel—possessed the utile traits of genius and longevity, such that there is an early, middle, and late Osler—each of which differs from the others. Years later, disciples and opponents alike can find plenty of fodder for whatever ideas suit them in the master's writings. What matters is not pulling a quote out of context but rather understanding where these thinkers came from, where they went, and how their ideas evolved.

This not being a book about Osler, let me refrain from an extensive review of his influence in later medical practice. I will pick out a few critiques, though, partly because they are directly germane to this book and partly because they come from the Rochester tradition of George Engel.[4]

One critique, as discussed above, is that Osler has little relevance to psychiatry because he was antipsychiatric, because he tended to focus reductionistically only on organic aspects of medicine. I have already discussed how this view is mistaken and ignores Osler's interest in neurasthenia and Weir's rest cure. One might add that, in his textbook and in his practice, Osler discussed extensively and paid great attention to the impact of psychological tension and stress on conditions like angina pectoris (Bliss 1999). Osler can be well defended against the oversimplified charge of reductionism.

A second critique comes from Engel himself; though without using Osler's name, it is clearly aimed at the Oslerian tradition:

> Most students have had among their mentors few models of truly scientific physicians. True, some are great clinical teachers, masterful in their clinical relationships and in their understanding of their patients, truly compassionate and humane physicians. However, their knowledge and skills in the human area derive largely from intuition, in part based on experience and in part based on innate personal characteristics. In many, it does not ever reach the cognitive level and therefore it can be neither communicated nor tested, hence the ready characterization as art rather than science. Such teachers are admired and emulated but cannot easily be learned from. They teach by precept and example, not by principles that can be identified or tested systematically. They espouse and exemplify humanism in medicine but they advance its scientific understanding little. And so it will remain until the need for a more inclusive scientific model for medicine is acknowledged, one that extends the scientific method to the human domain." (G. L. Engel 1987, p. 111)

Engel seems to want to put aside the entire apprenticeship aspect of medicine; four years of medical school are followed by four or more years of clinical apprenticeship (residency) because, contrary to Engel's view, book knowledge is not sufficient in medicine. Learning principles is not enough; one has to see good doctors in action, to see how they behave, what they do, and thus to *learn by example*. The process is little different from all kinds of behaviors that we learn as we grow from childhood into adulthood; children famously follow what their parents do, not what they say. Yet if Engel denigrates this teaching by example, it does not take much to find counterarguments. Perusal of *Muir's Thesaurus of Truths* (Muir and Muir 1937) produces Edmund Burke saying: "Example is the school of mankind; it will learn at no other." Or Seneca: "Men trust more to their eyes than to their ears. The effect of precepts is, therefore, slow and tedious, while that of examples is summary and effectual." Or William Ellery Channing: "Precept is instruction written in the sand . . . Example is graven on the rock" (all quotes p. 165). I'll stake my lot with Seneca and the gang. As for the reliance on "intuition" or "personal characteristics," Engel is ignoring another source, which he denigrates: the humanities themselves—literature and poetry and the arts, whose utility I will defend in the next chapter.

Despite valuing teaching by example, I also emphasize that this is not just about "intuition;" existential methods, which constitute much of the art of medicine, can be taught didactically. Leston Havens has written, for instance, a number of clinical books where he shows exactly how he practices such existential approaches when talking to patients (Havens 1985b, 1986, 1993, 1996). Empathy, for instance, might be seen as subjective and intuitive. But listen to Havens teach it didactically (Havens 1986). There are different aspects of empathy, he instructs: First, there is *motor empathy*. When the patient enters the room, I observe how he sits, how he stoops, his eye contact. Is he looking at me or at the floor? If he looks at me, I look at him. If he looks at the floor, I look at the floor. Eventually, if we both look at the floor long enough, he steals a glance at me, and I steal a glance at him. Then we go back to looking at the floor. Does he cross his legs? If so, I do; if not, I don't. Does he sit straight or lean to one side? I do the same. Soon, this nonverbal empathy establishes an unspoken sense of ease, of two similar people, rather than two opposed strangers. After motor empathy, Havens teaches that we should seek cognitive empathy: as the patient speaks, I try to match the thought patterns of the patient. Is he talking about sports? He mentions the Red Sox and how they have not done so well recently; I imagine that if I were talking about the Red Sox, I might discuss the recent injury to their star pitcher. Does he go there, or somewhere else? I try to think the patient's thoughts a split second before he thinks them; if I actually think he is going to say what he then says, then I have begun to establish cognitive empathy. After motor and cognitive empathy, one can then begin to feel *emotional empathy,* that aspect of empathy that is usually taken to be its meaning. Such emotional empathy flows from the hard work of motor and cognitive empathy, however; it does not just happen. It may seem like simple intuition to you, something that cannot be taught, but this is true only if you do not know what it is and do not know how to teach it.

A third critique of Osler is that he is irrelevant; this is the flip side of the first critique. There, Osler was the biological reductionist; here he is the clinical dilettante. One author puts it this way (Barondess 2002): "Some months ago at a medical meeting I heard a prominent academic, an expert in the application of electronic methods in medicine, announce that Oslerian medicine is dead. He meant low-tech medicine, medicine expressed especially in clinical sophistication at the bedside, coupled with masterful command of most of the content of the physician's field. . . . Interestingly, the audience understood, almost intuitively, what he meant." Has modern technology made Osler's clinical emphasis obsolete? Is Osler, the "historian-philosopher" an anachronism in the age of functional MRI? This critique is of course the biomedical reductionism that so exercised Engel and that led to the reaction of the BPS model. If indeed Oslerian medicine is dead, then perhaps Engel is right and the BPS model is a better alternative than pure biomedical reductionism. But Oslerian medicine need not be dead. It simply entails taking seriously the fact that the body that is diseased belongs to a human being who is a person. Put another way, "medicine, at its core, is oriented around the patient," who is a human being (Barondess 2002). (The author concludes that Oslerian medicine is still alive: "the pursuit of clinical excellence, in teaching, in lifelong scholarship, in connections with our traditions, and our forbears, in our devotion to each other and our best selves—all this was Osler's message" [Barondess 2002]). Because this basic fact will never go away, we must deal with it, and one avenue, one set of resources, lies in the humanities. That is the direction Osler took us, and, I suggest, it is the direction we need to resume, a path more effective and more profound than the BPS model.

One patient taught me this lesson well, when I was a medical intern, working on the cardiovascular unit at Massachusetts General Hospital. He was a 60-year-old former high school teacher, recovering from cardiac surgery. As I tended to the vital signs and chart, he became irritated: "You young doctors, you are all semi-educated. You know all about these tubes and tests, but I bet you don't know any Latin phrases." I turned back at the doorway to his room; he was looking at me with slight disdain, as if I was a student about to fail one of his pop quizzes. I searched my mind for any lost Latin phrase from the past. At last, one came to me, an ancient gladiator motto: *Moriturum te salutamus*,[5] I said triumphantly (though I mangled the conjugations). A faint smile came to his lips.

CHAPTER THIRTEEN

The Two Cultures

There is a natural hesitation and resistance against the humanities among scientifically oriented persons, many of whom choose to become physicians.[1] To them, the humanities seem not only foreign to, but also of unclear relevance to, medicine. They might even note that William Osler was neither a historian, nor a novelist, nor a poet, yet he acted the part in all these areas. And his exhortation to doctors to become humanistic, to read the Great Books—the Bible, Shakespeare, *Religio Medici,* and so on—all this may seem like mere nineteenth-century belles lettres, the views of an anachronistic Anglophile whose world disappeared with that same Great War that killed his only child.

Though stated callously, this critique is, at root: how does all this matter to medicine? We want to explain what is happening in the body, and yes, perhaps we want to understand the suffering of the individual human being who comes to us, but why all this biblical language and versification?

Robert Coles and the Call of Stories

By the written humanities, we mean literature, based on stories, and poetry, based on metaphor. So an appreciation for the humanities in medicine means appreciating stories and the power of metaphor. Let's begin with stories, a tradition well expressed by psychiatrist Robert Coles (1989).

As a young resident in the 1950s, Coles was anxious to translate patient's symptoms into theories, at that time psychoanalytic. Two supervisors contrasted. One kept trying to get him to interpret patients' experiences in terms of theory: "What are the psychodynamics at work here?" he kept pestering the young Coles (p. 6). The other urged him to listen to the stories people were telling him: "The people who come to see us bring us their stories. . . . They hope we know how to interpret their stories correctly." Coles reflected later: "He reminded me that psychiatrists often hover over their patients, intent on 'getting a fix' on them: make a diagnosis; ascertain what 'factors' or 'variables' have been at work; decide on a 'therapeutic agenda.' He wasn't criticizing such routine evaluative procedures, nor did he have any dramatic alternative to them. He simply wanted to remind me that I was hearing stories all day long." Here is the crux: Appreciation of patients' stories does not mean that we do not make diagnoses or treat them in a biomedical manner; it does mean that we understand that sometimes all of their stories can be interpreted biomedically, sometimes some of them, sometimes none. The stories are always the starting point and sometimes the ending as well.

And where can we learn to hear stories, to best interpret them, to best understand them? In the works of literature, in those classic old books by dead white men and also in newer books by multicolored authors. This realization led Coles to later teach a highly successful and prized course on medicine and literature at Harvard Medical School.

Coles was heavily influenced by two physician-writers, William Carlos Williams and Walker Percy. Williams, the poet who was a pediatrician, lived the life of a busy clinician and saw many kids, treating them biomedically. His appreciation for their humanity did not interfere with his medical abilities; it only made him a better physician:[2] "We have to pay the closest attention to what we say," Williams advised a young Coles. "What patients say tells us what to think about what hurts them; and what we say tells us what is happening to us—what we are thinking, and what may be wrong with us. . . . Their story, yours, mine—it's what we carry with us on this trip we take, and we owe it to each other to respect our stories and learn from them" (p. 30). In retrospect, Coles concludes: "Such a respect for narrative as everyone's rock-bottom capacity, but also as the universal gift, to be shared with others, seemed altogether fitting" (p. 30).

The Bible

To bring home the power of stories, let us think about one of the most powerful books ever written, or one might say, about one of the most influential persons in the world—the Bible. Now I do not say this based on any personal belief (I come from another tradition); I state it based as a fact that Christianity, along with Islam, is a major world religion, and that the two together comprise most of the world's population, and both give special credence to Jesus. It is famous, of course, that Christ spoke in parables, in stories. So too did Muhammad and Buddha. Jesus did not say: "You should treat each other equally." He said, "Love your neighbor as yourself." The two statements mean the same thing abstractly; but one uses metaphor, the other does not. Jesus would weave these metaphors into stories. He did not discuss altruism abstractly, but concretely, in the story of the Good Samaritan on the road to Jericho.

It is deeply human to have stories to tell, and if a physician takes seriously the notion that we must respect the patient as a person, as a human being, this can only mean to turn off our analytic minds, remove all theories from our thinking, to stop judging and interpreting, and to simply listen to the stories that people have to tell us. This gift, the "call of stories," is not given at birth, though, to most of us; like clinical and diagnostic skills, obtained only after years of practice, the skill of listening to stories is gained through years of practice in hearing stories (i.e., through intimate familiarity with humanistic literature).

Poetry and Metaphor

If literature is about stories, poetry is about metaphor. Nietzsche once said that truth is a mobile army of metaphors, and indeed it is. One might even argue, partially correctly, that most scientific concepts are also, at bottom, metaphor. Think of what it means when the neurobiologists say that transmission of memory is differentially "gated" in the amygdala, as opposed to the neocortex, for emotional content. Or when we talk about Heisenberg's uncertainty principle, and we picture photons of light "hitting" spheric atoms (Okasha 2002). Physicist Richard Feynman knew about the centrality of visual imagery to scientific thinking: "When I see equations, I see the letters in colors—I don't know why. As I'm talking, I see vague pictures of Bessel functions . . . with light—tan j's, slightly violet-bluish n's, and dark brown x's flying around. And I wonder what the hell it must look like to the students" (Feynman 1988, p. 59). Visual and verbal metaphors abound in much scientific work. (This is not to say that some science, like pure algebra, can be "image-less," though Feynman's experience throws doubt on even that notion.)

As human beings wishing to know, our options are not metaphors versus facts, literature versus science, but one kind of metaphor versus another kind of metaphor. Once we recognize that science too operates with metaphors, disguised in abstract language no doubt but still metaphors, then the value of poetry cannot be dismissed out of hand.[3]

Borges on Poetry

Argentine poet Jorge Luis Borges, blind and near the end of his life, gave a series of lectures at Harvard that brought out the essential nature of poetry (Borges 2000). A key point to his thinking was that not only is metaphor essential to poetry, but so is also all language, all words: all knowledge is dependent on metaphor.

"Life is, I am sure, made of poetry," Borges began, noting that poetry grows out of the subjective experience of humans: "Bishop Berkeley said that the taste of the apple is neither in the apple itself—the apple cannot taste itself—nor in the mouth of the eater. It requires contact between them" (p. 3). He went on to emphasize that poetry taps into fundamental aspects of our existence: "We know what poetry is. We know it so well that we cannot define it in the other words, even as we cannot define the taste of coffee, the color red or yellow, or the meaning of anger, of love of hatred, of the sunrise, of the sunset, of our love of country" (p. 17).

He then got to the key role of metaphor: "Argentine poet Leopoldo Lugones said that every word is a dead metaphor. You will find the metaphor tucked away somewhere in the etymology of every word" (p. 22). Thus, metaphor is not something extra, or something avoidable; it is at the root of all language, all verbal communication. And the power of metaphor, Borges said, is that "anything suggested is far more effective than anything laid down" (p. 31). Metaphors tend to be concrete images, usually visual, that correspond to the natural world. Though Borges did not make this point, one might speculate that such visual, sensual imagery taps into the evolutionary roots of language, thus affecting our thinking more effectively and more profoundly than abstract thought. In other words, the brain might be more adapted to metaphorical thinking—like poetry—than to abstract thinking—like science. Borges approximates this line of thought: "Words began not by being abstract, but rather by being concrete. . . . Thus poetry is bringing language back to its original source" (pp. 79–80).

If my speculation about the evolutionary role of metaphor is valid, it dovetails with an interesting and original aspect of Borges's lectures—his claim that there are only a few basic metaphors, the many combinations of which represent the uniqueness of poetic creativity. "Only a dozen or so patterns of metaphor exist . . . but those patterns are capable of almost endless variations" (p. 21). These basic metaphors include the analogy of eyes to stars, of women to flowers, of time to rivers, of life to dreaming, of death to sleeping, and of fire to battles (pp. 32–33; Borges provided many examples in verse).

Borges pointed out that distrust of metaphor is behind most denigration of poetry: "Our idea of words' being a mere algebra of symbols comes from dictionaries. . . . Having long catalogues of words and explanations makes us think that the explanations exhaust the words. . . . But every word stands by itself. . . . Every word is unique" (p. 91). Borges feels in fact that we are unable to express ourselves without metaphor, that all communication is ultimately metaphorical, and thus that poetry is merely an attempt to communicate as well as possible using metaphors: "I no longer believe in expression; I believe only in *allusion*. After all, what are words? *Words are symbols for shared memories*. If I use a word, then you should have some experience of what the word stands for. . . . If not, the word means nothing to you. I think we can only allude, we can only try to make the reader imagine" (p. 117, italics in original).

Beyond the central role of metaphor, Borges also felt that the experience of the meaning of poetry is not just an intellectual exercise; rather, like Wilhelm Dilthey (see chapter 15), he held that such understanding grew out of combining rational thought with other aspects of our mind, particularly our emotions and our will: "We *feel* the beauty of a poem before we even begin to think of a meaning" (p. 84, italics in original). Others have emphasized that poetry is based on intuition as a source of knowledge, rather than sense-data or empirical observation (Ros-Janet 2005). If we accept that external sense-data are not the only source of knowledge, then first-person subjective experience seems relevant to human knowledge (the "taste" of the apple). Poetry may be relevant in recruiting these other aspects of mental life.

In sum, Borges teaches us two key features of poetry: the central role of metaphor and the impact of other aspects of our mental make-up besides intellect—particularly emotions and will. Both of these features may tie into our evolutionary heritage: All words began as metaphors, as concrete and often visual depictions, because our language originated, in the mists of evolution, in response to the concrete natural world. Poetry is faithful to the origin of language and returns us to its roots. Intellect and rationality, a late evolutionary achievement, was long preceded by emotions and by action. By recruiting emotions and will, poetry takes us back to our deeper mental heritage; it brings forth our whole being, not just gray theory (as Goethe put it) but the green realities of our feelings and wishes and desires and actions—our whole being.

If we appreciate these two features of poetry, which can be extended to all literature, then we can appreciate that the humanities—poetry and literature—are not optional, not an accessory that we can live with or without, nor a fluffy obsession with words that adds nothing to real science but rather the core of life itself.[4]

Max Eastman's *Enjoyment of Poetry*

In his book *Enjoyment of Poetry* (Eastman 1921), American socialist intellectual Max Eastman speculates about a metaphor for life: suppose we are all passengers on a ferry, leaving one harbor to go to another. He imagines that two kinds of persons could be identified: those who come to the ferry stern, looking around, smelling the wind, enjoying the air; and those who move into the belly of the ship, to converse, to drink, to smoke, and perhaps to nap. The first is the poetic person, interested in the ride; the second is the practical person, focused on the destination. We humans are partly both, Eastman says, but one or the other kind (the poetic or the practical) predominates in each of us.

Eastman is picking out something about the poetic predisposition that removes it from the world of fantasy and brings it into the very nature of humanity: the poetic "wish to experience life and the world. That is the essence of the poetic temper" (p. 6).

He emphasizes the deeply common and human nature of the poetic temperament by describing how we are all this way during childhood: "Children are poetic. They love the feel of things. . . . They are not practical. They have not yet felt the necessity, or got addicted to the trick, of formulating a purpose and then achieving it. . . . It is easy for children to taste the qualities of experience, because experience is new. . . . Each [thing] is concrete, particular, unique, and without any habitual use" (pp. 6–7). One thinks of the wise words of the Italian poet Giacomo Leopardi: "Children see everything in nothing; grown-ups see nothing in everything" (Leopardi 1983). My five-year-old son recently was scratched by a plant with thorns: he labeled it the "spikybush"—he is a poet.

As we grow older, and get adapted to the world of everyday life, we lose our childhood curiosity—that sense of wonder that Einstein labeled as the ultimate source of all knowledge, including science.

This poetic origin to our existence never completely disappears; it gets reflected in how we label and understand the world around us. Just as there are poetic and practical *temperaments,* writes Eastman, we give poetic and practical *names* to all the things around us. The practical names "indicate a suitable adjustment" to things, the poetic names "engender a strong realization" of things (p. 22). "The conversation of the poetic is acute and exhilarating, waking you to the life and eminence in reality of all things. The conversation of the practical is instructive, interesting, sometimes full of surprise and a feeling of supreme possibility" (p. 30). The practical approach, purified and maximized, is science.

We know the distinction between poetic and practical names; it fills our language. In English, especially, the poetic names tend to be more Anglo-Saxon, the practical more Latin. Sometimes they are clearly set side by side, as in books of botany or guides to ornithology: Eastman would have us "imagine two people walking in leisure . . . along the roadside. It is summer and the yellow-birds are holding their sprightly revels among the milkweed blossoms there, dancing along before them as they go. 'Regular little *butterflies,* aren't they?' says one. 'Yes,' says the other faintly, and then, with emphasis: 'It is the *American goldfinch,* you know—a *grosbeak*'" (p. 31, all italics in original). Comparing books of botany and ornithology, Eastman claims the opposition of the poetic and the practical is most clearly laid out: "There, side by side, you may read them—on the one line, labels picked from a language whose poetry is dead, and applied by earnest minds to serve the business of intellectual manipulation and accurate reference, and, on the other line, names bestowed in living syllables by the hearts of rural people in happy moments of carefree and vivid experience. Trailing Arbutus, Bouncing Bet, Dragon's Blood, Beggar's Buttons, Nose-bleed, Gay Feather, Heart-o'-the-earth, Ruby-throat, Fire-tail, Hell Diver, Solitary Vireo, Vesper Sparrow—these are the words for those who care but to feel and celebrate the qualities of things" (p. 32).

We see this everywhere "and, in the lavish persistence, and in the truth, of these meadow names, holding their own against so much Latin, there is a lesson in humility for all science." For, after all, which is the right name: "water" or "H_2O"? Is one correct, and the other wrong? If there is no role for poetry or the humanities in human existence, then "water" must be wrong. Yet "H_2O" does not provide the same meaning to us that "water" does. Eastman's point (like that of Dilthey later) is that one name is not right nor the other wrong, nor is there one world in which that thing is water and another world in which it is H_2O. It is "water" everywhere. What differs is not the thing itself; what differs is our purposes, what we, as human beings, want to achieve or say or appreciate. If we wish to conduct an experiment of organic chemistry, "H$_2$O" will do; if we want to wash our hands, "water" works. The poetic has a role in life, side by side with the practical.

Eastman also touches on the same key point as Borges about the metaphorical roots of all words and adds examples, showing how the etymology of words reveals their concrete poetic roots: "*Gymnasium,* 'the place of nakedness' . . . *Sarcasm,* 'flesh-tearing' . . . [The poet] has called men *half-baked* also, at least *cooked too quick* in the word *precocious;* and the word *delirious* he has called them, not *off their trolley,* but what is the same thing in an earlier state of civilization, *out of their furrow*" (p. 57, all italics in original). Eastman expands this source of poetry from metaphor, which has a narrow literary meaning, to the broader idea that poetic language involves comparison of some kind or another, based on a choice made by the poet. This comparison can be by analogy, by simile, by metaphor, by sound, by rhythm, and so on, but comparison, of some kind, with some chosen concrete quality, makes it poetry.

Poetry and Individuality

So Eastman provides a further justification of poetry that he relates to human nature, to the essentially experiential temperament of children, and to the qualitative concrete aspect of naming words. He further holds, like Borges, that poetic language is at the root of all words.[5]

He is not unaware of claims otherwise. Indeed, writing in the early twentieth century, at the end of the Victorian era of progress and science, and before the disillusionment of two world wars, Eastman was writing against that simplistic positivism in science that Dilthey and others resisted (see chapter 15). He knew there was another view. Even a poet as great as Percy Shelley could see it: "The deep truth is imageless," he said (Eastman 1921, p. 140). Could it be that the concrete roots of poetic language were, after all, primitive, and bound to be eliminated by the progress of science? Could we ever have a fully imageless abstract knowledge? One might suppose that mathematics represented such, or perhaps symbolic logic. Did such fields represent the surpassing of poetry?

Eastman tried to answer by examining the debate raging within science and philosophy between the positivists and the nonpositivists; he took up the concept of two types of knowing: the explanation of general concepts or laws versus the understanding of concrete individual realities (which I discuss in detail in the next chapter and the appendix). Poetry, he argued, as have many others, reflects the individual unique realities of life. So even though purely abstract general knowledge can exist, as in mathematics and logic, it does not capture other aspects of knowledge, namely, that of the particular and unique: "The world does not exist in the abstract, nor in general, nor in any classification, but in concrete and heterogeneous detail. The poet reminds us of this. Poetry is a countryman, and greets every experience by its own name" (p. 147).

This sense of the concreteness of poetry was beautifully expressed by William Carlos Williams (1983), when he spoke of the mission of poetry as involving "No ideas / but in things." Williams taught us that metaphor allows a reconciliation between "the people and the stones." Compose, he advised the poet within each of us; ideas and stones are not all that different.

No ideas but in things—there we have the essential philosophy of poetry.[6]

And then there is the world of emotion. Mathematics and logic is all about . . . logic. But the human mind is only partly logic and reason; neocortex sits atop paleocortex, frontal inhibition above limbic fight-or-flight. The world of poetry touches our experience of emotion in a way general science never approaches. Here is Eastman's example of what he describes as "the passion and its images" in a great poem:

Remember me when I am gone away,
Gone far away into the silent land;
When you can no more hold me by the hand,
Nor I half turn to go yet turning stay.
Yet if you should forget me for a while
And afterwards remember, do not grieve;
For if the darkness and corruption leave
A vestige of the thoughts that once I had,
Better by far you should forget and smile
Than that you should remember and be sad. (p. 165)

I might add a poem by Mary E. Frye for the dead, rich in metaphor as well as emotion:

Do not stand at my grave and weep,
I am not there. I do not sleep.
I am a thousand winds that blow,
I am the diamond glints on snow.
I am the sunlight on ripened grain.

I am the gentle autumn rain.
When you awake in the morning's hush,
I am the swift uplifting rush
Of quiet birds in circling flight.
I am the soft starshine at night.
Do not stand at my grave and cry,
I am not there. I did not die.

Four Pillars of Poetry

Eastman shows us two more features of poetry (besides its link to human nature and its reflection of the etymology of words): poetry captures the concrete, the real, the unique; and poetry connects to human emotion. These last two aspects of poetry are what some philosophers (like Dilthey) would see as central to knowledge of human beings.

Eastman was aware that his generalizations about poetry as a whole did not capture differences within the world of poetry; some promote free verse, others emphasize rhyme. Edgar Allan Poe defined poetry as "a pleasurable idea accompanied by music" (p. 247); some focus on the concrete and everyday (like Walt Whitman), others on expression of emotion (like Poe). But these differences occur within a larger context—the value of the poetic as part of human nature, essential to human language, and faithful to concrete experience.

The Two Cultures

The arguments of Eastman, and later of Borges, did not stem the divergent evolution of the Western intellect, what Cambridge scholar C. P. Snow would come to call, in a celebrated 1959 lecture, "the two cultures" of science and the humanities (Snow 1993). Snow was initially trained in science and worked for a while in experimental physics, but mainly considered himself a novelist. When invited to give the prestigious Gifford Lectures, he gave a talk that generated commentary and criticism for decades. Yet Snow did not seek to defend the humanities from science; rather, he was arguing for the reverse. He saw a nonscientific world of academia, literature, and politics, in which scientific knowledge was limited, to the detriment of humanity.

Snow wanted to bring about a reconciliation, one that recognized differing strengths. Instead he saw two cultures of distrust: "The non-scientists have a rooted impression that the scientists are shallowly optimistic, unaware of man's condition. On the other hand, the scientists believe that the literary intellectuals are totally lacking in foresight, peculiarly unconcerned with their brother-men, in a deep sense anti-intellectual, anxious to restrict both art and thought to the existential moment" (p. 5). He comments that literary intellectuals—his term for those in the world of the humanities—view scientists as "brash and boastful," superficial advocates of technology who do not appreciate the pathos of existence. Snow notes that his scientist friends are all too aware of the fact that "the individual condition of each of us is tragic. Each of us is alone. . . . But nearly all of them . . . would see no reason why just because the individual condition is tragic, so must the social condition be." Scientists tend to be more socially optimistic, willing to try to use technology to improve the human lot, whether it be by curing medical disease or through reducing famine and hunger.

These are debates between two cultures, one of which might as well come from the sands of Arabia, the other from the shores of Iceland. These two cultures are bound to misinterpret each other, partly because there are few translators who can speak to both. The concept of two cultures is, says Snow, "a little more than a dashing metaphor, a good deal less than a cultural map."[7] Whatever its limits, the metaphor of two cultures highlights how these differences are, in some sense, expectable, but also ameliorable.

We can expect the differences, but we need to avoid demeaning and devaluing the other side: "The polarisation is sheer loss to us all." Both sides are "self-impoverished" because they ignore the other; they are "tone-deaf" to each other: "As with the tone-deaf, they don't know what they miss" (p. 14). In particular, Snow wants to shake the literary intellectuals out of their sense of know-it-all complacency: "A good many times I have been present at gatherings of people who, by the standards of the traditional culture, are thought highly educated and who have with considerable gusto been expressing their incredulity at the illiteracy of scientists. Once or twice I have been provoked and have asked the company how many of them could describe the Second Law of Thermodynamics. The response was cold: it was also negative. Yet I was asking something which is about the scientific equivalent of: *Have you read a work of Shakespeare's?*" (italics in original, pp. 15–16). Snow later averred that perhaps his choice of that physical law was not the best scientific example, for it could be criticized as a hypothesis rather than a scientific fact or discovery. Nonetheless, his point was made: there is such a thing as unacceptable scientific ignorance, and most nonscientists, even the most intellectual among them, are ignorant scientifically. Snow's larger point was that this ignorance was not a technical matter, but rather, in a world of atomic bombs and colonialism and famine (and, we might add today, the human genome project and stem cell research), such scientific ignorance on the part of the intellectual elite (not to mention the masses) is dangerous.

He later wrote: "I now believe that if I had asked an even simpler question— such as, What do you mean by mass, or acceleration, which is the scientific equivalent of saying, *Can you read?*—not more than one in ten of the highly educated would have felt that I was speaking the same language. So the great edifice of modern physics goes up, and the majority of the cleverest people in the western world have about as much insight into it as their Neolithic ancestors would have had" (p. 15, italics in original).

Snow went on to criticize educational systems, especially in Britain, that aim students toward either the sciences or the humanities to the exclusion of the other. He pointed out how the scientific revolution was at the root of the industrial revolution, and that antiscience humanists were "natural Luddites," failing to understand the basic motor of the modern world. He emphasized that major progress in basic problems in the world—especially disease and hunger—could be made with further scientific advances, but only if political and literary intellectuals appreciated the role and potential of science. "Closing the gap between our cultures," he concluded, "is a necessity in the most abstract intellectual sense, as well as in the most practical. . . . Isn't it time we began? The danger is, we have been brought up to think as though we had all the time in the world. We have very little time. So little that I dare not guess at it" (pp. 50–51).

Snow's critique was aimed at doyens of the humanities, dismissive of the sciences, stuck in a world that had long been left behind by the industrial revolution. My critique is directed at the scientists, especially in my field of medicine and psychiatry, dismissive of the humanities, creating a barren world where humanity is boxed up in categories and definitions, and human beings are nowhere to be seen. From both directions, the two cultures need to reconcile.

Taking Words Seriously

So we have here the witness of three wise men of the humanities: Borges, Eastman, Snow. They remind us that human beings mainly communicate by words (though partly too, like animals, nonverbally). All culture, and all science too, involves symbols (sometimes mathematics, usually words). All thought involves words, at some level. If we want to take culture and science seriously, then we have to take words seriously. And if they are right, and words are at root metaphorical, then we might say that poetry is a kind of *science of words,* in the Aristotelian notion of science (different from my definition in the glossary), meaning a discipline that is appropriate to its content. Poetry is essential to using words, appreciating language and communication, and thus understanding human beings.

Human beings think with their reason and intellect (the neocortex), but they also have feelings and emotions, and they will and act (with their paleocortex). The humanities speak to the whole mind, not just part of it.

If Engel or others want to dispense with poetry and the humanities, they have to provide better avenues for human communication with words, and they have to explain how we can better involve the emotions and the will in our models of medicine and psychiatry.[8]

Stories and Metaphors

All great literature is composed of stories and metaphors that speak through millennia. The content of this literature over human history has been similar. Homer tells the story of war and trauma, much as is experienced today by our own soldiers (Shay 1995). The human condition has changed, and it has stayed the same. The frequency and kinds of illnesses that we contract have changed. The plague is replaced by AIDS and pneumonia by cancer, and prevention of early childhood illness is replaced with concerns about childhood obesity. Yet, while postponed, death still happens, we come to this world and we go, with parents and siblings, growing up to love another person, experience sex, have children, succumb to disease, and sometimes kill each other in war. These facts of human history are the same now as ever, though with some variations in time and culture. It is to these human facts that literature returns again and again. And it is these themes that go to that special part of our human nature that no other type of knowledge seems to touch. Science, wonderful as it is, cannot tell us how to react to disease or death, nor does it explain why we kill or love. It can provide some knowledge in those fields, as it does elsewhere, but it fails to provide all we need to know (as positivism would wish).

To sum up, if metaphor and stories are so central to human life, then we should expect that they would be relevant to medicine and psychiatry. Susan Sontag perhaps most famously made the connection between metaphor and medicine (Sontag 1978). She focused on culturally important illnesses, like tuberculosis and cancer. Her point was not that these conditions could not, and should not, be conceived biologically within a standard medical model, but that they *also* had strong cultural connotations. Psychiatrist Ronald Pies also discussed the role of metaphor in psychiatric practice, emphasizing how metaphors can both help and hinder clinical treatment (Pies 2007). For instance, if a medication is viewed as a "crutch," the negative connotations of the metaphor are more likely to lead to noncompliance than if medication is described as a "bridge" toward better health or recovery. We might add the ideas of psychiatrist Leston Havens about "performative language" (a notion derived from philosopher J. L. Austin; (Austin 1975; Havens 1986, 1994). Havens was interested in the fact that some words are not *mere* words; they actually *do* things. To use Austin's lingo, descriptive phrases only depict something; performative phrases enact something. Thus, when the bride and groom say "I do," those phrases change their lives forever. Havens wondered whether effective psychotherapy might not be a species of performative language (Ghaemi 1999). All this rich tradition and creative thinking would seem to lead to only one conclusion: medicine and psychiatry dare not dispense with the power of words—with the humanities—too lightly.

A Story

We can end, appropriately, with a story. In 1989, as a visiting medical student in London, I followed a neurologist at King's College Hospital. During morning appointments, five British medical students joined me behind our professor; while he sat at his desk, patients would enter one by one. One day, during a break between patients, he turned to us and asked, "Who can recite a poem to me?" No one could (or perhaps dared). He turned, disgusted, and remarked, "How can you expect to be good doctors if you know no poetry?" He taught me that day the basic lesson of medical humanism—science is not enough to be a good physician; because we deal with persons and not just bodies, we need to relate to individual human beings, and the best repository of that knowledge lies in the humanities.

Perhaps Hippocrates and Osler had it right: we do not need a new model (hardheaded though psychological); we need to recover an old model, never fully realized, first brought forward by that ancient Greek from Cos, lost under centuries of dust and dogma, briefly revived by Osler, that Canadian lover of all things ancient, but again pushed aside in the name of the locomotive and the couch.

CHAPTER FOURTEEN

Between Science and the Humanities

The debate between science and the humanities gets at the core of the philosophical problem underlying the biopsychosocial (BPS) model: Is science, valuable as it is, the main road to knowledge? If not, how is the method of the humanities different? This philosophical problem lands us in the real world of the practicing psychiatrist and psychologist. Should we be dualists, with two approaches to the mind and body, or monists, or pluralists, or eclectics?

We need to answer this question if we are to have a coherent conception of what we are doing. The BPS model sought to reply differently from either biological psychiatry or traditional psychoanalysis. Or perhaps it is simply a way of avoiding a reply.

But answer we must, and, because medicine can harm as well as help, we must answer correctly.

Ways of Knowing

A complex and lengthy literature on science and the humanities, dating back over a century, awaits us. We might begin to approach it by noting two basic views: the idea that there is only one way of knowing versus the view that there are two or more. One view holds that all knowledge is of one kind; in the hands of positivists, the belief is that all knowledge is, or will become, scientific. This might be called the "consilience" model, the idea that all fields of knowledge ultimately lead to a unified science (Wilson 1999). Sociology will become sociobiology, psychology will become cognitive science, and so on. The other view holds that there is a fundamental difference between natural and human sciences—the "two cultures" model —that the two approaches at a basic level cannot be equalized. Thus, we have H_2O —three atoms connected chemically—and we have water—a liquid substance that runs over my hand a certain way. They are two different ways of knowing; one cannot replace the other.

If this second view is correct, then we need to understand humanistic knowledge, how it differs from science, and how we can apply, teach, and practice it in psychiatry. In chapter 15, I trace this debate in more philosophical detail. Here I will summarize my conclusions as related to the BPS model.

Psychiatric Pluralism: The Rejection of Dogmatism and Eclecticism

Many of us go through life assuming that there is only one kind of knowledge and many kinds of error. You can be right only one way; everything else is wrong. This would seem to be common sense, and ever since Sunday school, we are imbued in our bones with this assumption. Some of us have been infected with the theories of Michel Foucault, though we might never have read him; one finds this infection in the adolescent who says that what *is* good is what *feels* good; that every person is the judge of his or her own morality; and that everything is relative.[1]

Either there is only one knowledge or there is no knowledge: This is where most of us are in our own personal philosophies. Among believers in only one kind of knowledge, we find two subsets, roughly equal in number. The first believe that all knowledge is scientific; for them, the touchstone of everything is experience and experiment. If you can put a number on it, they are happy; if you can add a statistical *p*-value, they are ecstatic. The second believe that all knowledge is metaphysical; usually religious, sometimes secular. Here one finds the mass of humankind in their deepest beliefs: a faith in another world, a God or gods, books of revelation, Ten Commandments, reincarnation, a chosen people. These two groups are less in conflict than they imagine. It could be that all this back and forth between atheists and believers, scientists and philosophers is nothing more than category errors in both camps. Perhaps the ways of science are irrelevant to the world of faith and vice versa.

In other words, many people are dogmatists: they believe in religion and nothing else; or they believe in science and nothing else. I am not claiming that most people are this way, nor am I proving that this is the case. But the history of humankind should provide sufficient evidence that many dogmatists have existed, and continue to exist, in human societies.

Beyond dogmatism, there is another possibility: perhaps there are two kinds of knowledge—or twenty—each of them valid in its own realm. This would be one definition of the term *pluralism* (see glossary). This is not relativism; each kind of knowledge is not equally valid, nor should they be mixed up: don't bother consulting the Talmud to understand the Krebs cycle in cells; don't try to use the second law of thermodynamics to explain the creation of Adam. No, method-based pluralism is not relativism, it is not eclecticism, it does not license adolescent libertinism. It is democratic, hemmed in by laws and responsibilities on all sides, a source of guidance that rejects the tyranny of dogma as well as the anarchy of eclecticism.

The Triad of *Verstehen:* A Method-Based Psychiatry

Let me simplify: there is not one approach to knowledge (be it scientific versus religious); there is no absolutely valid knowledge; there are two or more valid approaches to knowledge, as long as they are applied predominantly in their own fields.

This is the core of the pluralist philosophy (when stripped of relativist and postmodernist misinterpretations; a better term may be *method-based psychiatry*). It is the core of the best alternative to biopsychosocial eclecticism in medicine and psychiatry.

Many prominent proponents of the method-based model have argued for two basic approaches to knowledge. I must import two German words, for which, the German original seems more accurate and practical for future discussion. The two approaches to knowledge are *Erklären* (causal explanation) and *Verstehen* (meaningful understanding).[2]

Erklären is commonly understood as science (though it is only partly so, in fact). It is objective and empirical and based on external experience. It proceeds by experiment and is replicable, able to be falsified or confirmed by independent scientists. This is the view of knowledge that many in our modern scientific age automatically assume represents the only true or real form of knowledge. The method-based perspective grants validity to *Erklären* but limits its scope. *Erklären* is most valid for the natural sciences—for biology and chemistry and physics. For the humanities and the human sciences—for religion and sociology and psychology and philosophy and literature and poetry—it has less utility. There is another approach to knowledge, on this view: *Verstehen.* (Most of my exposition will work off of the version of *Verstehen* propounded by the nineteenth-century German philosopher Wilhelm Dilthey.)

The first approximation to *Verstehen* is to emphasize the first-person perspective, contrasting with the third-person in *Erklären; Verstehen* is mostly subjective; *Erklären* mostly objective. This is not all there is to *Verstehen,* because it also involves, as noted below, external observation of the expressions and statements of others, but this subjectivity is a key feature. It is especially relevant to psychiatry, because we deal with mental states as our primary phenomena of study. If we accept that mental states are inherently subjective and occur to another person whom we seek to understand, then the first-person perspective of that person would appear relevant. This problem of "other minds" is the source of intense philosophical debate. Most would agree, though, that mental states occur in the private world of our feelings and desires and that much of the work of psychiatry involves getting to know these mental states.

The next feature of *Verstehen* is described by Dilthey as follows: "Understanding [*Verstehen*] we call the process by which mental life comes to be known through an expression of it given to the senses" (Rickman 1988). Dilthey is trying to emphasize here that *Verstehen* is not mysterious but an extension of common sense. Just as one of our approaches to knowledge has to do with natural objects (which we observe externally and empirically based on our five senses and technological extensions of those senses, such as microscopes, telescopes, MRIs), we have another kind of knowledge that has to do with what human beings say and how they behave (with the verbal and nonverbal expressions of human beings usually reflecting the internal mental states of those humans: their feelings, beliefs, judgments, wishes, and intentions). At some level, then, *Verstehen* involves behavioral and observable inferences about what philosophers call "intentionality," the wish to do things.[3]

Another aspect to *Verstehen* is the sense of meaning. *Verstehen* involves creating or discovering a meaning for a phenomenon, based not solely on the first-person experience of a person, but, rather, on an overall understanding obtained through research about that phenomenon. The human phenomenon (say, auditory hallucinations) is studied, empathized with in the first person, analyzed empirically in the third person, examined with recourse to its relations to other human phenomena (e.g., cultural features), and then the researcher comes up with a synthetic meaning for the whole.[4]

Thus, there is a triad of features to *Verstehen*: subjective experience, verbal and nonverbal expressions, and meaning-creation.[5] I will expand on this description in the next chapter.

Engel's Mix

We are now at the conceptual core of the BPS model.

If pluralism—a method-based approach to knowledge—is false, if *Erklären* suffices for all knowledge, then there is no need for a BPS model. Pure biological psychiatry will do. There is no need for anything in medicine but tests, cold, hard steel (as in surgery), and drugs. (Further, we can stop teaching Shakespeare and just focus on mathematics instead; indeed, some would hold, not unjustifiably, that this process has happened in the "closing of the American mind" [Bloom 1988].)

The BPS movement was an implicit recognition that this purely positivistic perspective on the world is mistaken. The question is: what else is there?

By now it should be obvious that there are the humanities and the social sciences, disciplines that involve human beings. German literature dubs them *Geisteswissenschaften*—literally translated as "sciences of the spirit" but used to mean "human sciences." Some use the term *human studies* (see chapter 15). There is poetry and literature and history and sociology and anthropology and political science and economics. Unless we want to throw all these disciplines in the trash, it would seem that we need to find a place for them in any general theory of knowledge, and, in medicine and psychiatry, we need to identify how they apply to our work.

The terms *Verstehen* and *Erklären* are ways of trying to organize all these disciplines based on showing how these two cognitive processes are best used: Most of the natural and physical sciences use *Erklären*, and some of the social sciences do (e.g., mathematical analyses of public spending in economics); most of the humanities and social sciences use *Verstehen*, and some of the natural sciences do (e.g., biological research on animal behavior).

Medicine, and in particular its subdiscipline of psychiatry, would seem to be exactly in the middle of all these fields, smack dab in the middle on the spectrum of *Erklären* and *Verstehen*. We use both.

The BPS model was an attempt to capture this special fact, but it did so without clear conceptual analysis and without the proper philosophical context. To the extent that it tried to provide any conceptual justification, it alluded to the need for holism (as in general systems theory). But this general appeal to holism is vague and nonspecific. In practice, as we have seen, the BPS model was eclecticism, a willingness to mix and match, as one wished, *Verstehen* and *Erklären* to one's liking. Yet within medicine and psychiatry, there are places for mostly *Erklären*, and places for mostly *Verstehen*, and sometimes both—but not always both and not always whichever one prefers.

Some of this lack of conceptual clarity has to do with the fact that George Engel explicitly (and Roy Grinker implicitly) rejected any distinction to be made between *Erklären* and *Verstehen*. For them, there was only one form of knowledge: empirical science—*Erklären*. All Engel was saying was that we needed to augment the *Erklären* of biological science with the *Erklären* of psychological and social sciences.[6] One might be more generous and grant that Engel allowed some *Verstehen* in his BPS model, but it was still an approach to meaning that relied on only two main sources, psychology and sociology. Engel left out many other cultural sources of *Verstehen*-based knowledge. For all the attraction the BPS model appears to possess for humanistically oriented types in the mental health professions, he specifically excluded the humanities.

The Scope of *Verstehen*

If we reject the BPS model and if we reject sole reliance on *Erklären*, the next question is what kind of *Verstehen* will we allow into our understanding of medicine and psychiatry, and, perhaps as importantly, how would it play out in practice?

First we must address the scope of *Verstehen*. Is it just the humanities, just the social sciences, or both? And how are we to understand that German term *Geisteswissenschaften* (the human studies)? (I will limit myself in this discussion to relevance to medicine and psychiatry.)

Those who have most prominently discussed this question in modern American psychiatry, Paul McHugh and Phillip Slavney at the Johns Hopkins University, have tended to focus on *Verstehen* as a method of logical reasoning (as an epistemological method, a way of knowing; Slavney and McHugh 1987): "Explanation is no more 'fundamental' than understanding, nor is understanding more 'profound' than explanation; they are only different methods, with different strengths and weaknesses. As long as we continue to view human beings as object/organisms *and* subject/agents, both methods are essential to our practice." Unfortunately, despite their warnings and their critiques of the BPS model, this method-based view of psychiatry presented by Slavney and McHugh is too often interpreted eclectically: See, concludes the novice looking for a rationale for continuing to believe in whatever psychological theory appeals to him, everything is not just biology (Muller 2008). Well, that is true, but one has to know when matters are mostly biological, and when they are not, and why so. Glib assumptions that all methods are appropriate are based on a failure to understand the meaning and uses of *Erklären* and *Verstehen*. Slavney and McHugh make *Verstehen* a primarily cognitive technique (much as in the tradition of Max Weber, see next chapter) and thus, in their many works, they can be read as emphasizing the social sciences over the humanities (although elsewhere McHugh emphasizes the importance of the humanities).[7]

Another perspective, however, is found in the work of Dilthey (Makkreel 1991, 1992). His view was that the concept of *Verstehen* is not purely logical. Rather it also involves intuition and emotion and the use of all aspects of one's being: "We explain through purely intellectual processes, but we understand through the cooperation of all our mental powers" (Ermarth 1978, p. 246). For Dilthey, the distinction between *Erklären* and *Verstehen* was a distinction between two ways of being-in-the-world, two types of worldview (*Weltanschauung*), two approaches to life. Though they are different kinds of logic, these approaches cannot be purely reduced to simple logic; they are also different ways of being, different totalities of how to understand and live in the world. In this sense, *Verstehen* is an ontological concept, as philosophers would put; it involves one's being—one's emotions and will, not just one's ideas or thoughts. This is why Dilthey talked about his viewpoint as being the "philosophy of life," an appreciation of the real flow of life, not just abstractions from sense-data as in positivism. It is not that "thought grasps life"; "life grasps life," based on augmentation of intellect with our feelings or emotions and our actions (Rickman 1988, p. 134). As such, *Verstehen* would thus apply not just to intellectual activities—like the social sciences—but also to emotional or intuitive activities—like poetry and the humanities. Indeed, in an extensive but unsystematic corpus of writings, Dilthey included a treatise on poetics, highlighting how important he felt poetry was to human experience (Dilthey 1985). He also was musically trained and saw music as essential to being human (Ermarth 1978). As neurologist Michael Trimble has suggested, perhaps the brain is the best synthesizer of *Erklären* and *Verstehen*, for it seems equally adapted for higher logic and music (Trimble 2007).

A Theory of Knowledge

In agreement with McHugh and Slavney, and in contrast to Engel, we need to appreciate *Verstehen* and *Erklären* in psychiatry and medicine. It is important to understand that *Verstehen* and *Erklären* are not just different methods, or different *kinds* of knowledge, but different *aspects* of all knowledge. Together, they provide a full and valid appreciation of science. In a way, following Dilthey, *Verstehen* and *Erklären* should be seen as two ends of a spectrum, not as two completely separate and opposite categories. All knowledge moves along this spectrum, sometimes more as *Erklären*, sometimes more as *Verstehen*, occasionally it sits in the middle, using both. Perhaps all views are partially correct in this old debate: all knowledge is one, but it has two aspects. In that case, Osler was right: we need to appreciate *Verstehen* explicitly (and perhaps even primarily) as represented in the humanities, not just the social or psychological sciences.

Here, then, may be the best avenue to go beyond the BPS model, while also rejecting psychiatric dogmatisms: we need to move to a method-based psychiatry, which entails being more clear about our methods.

CHAPTER FIFTEEN

The Meaning of Meaning

Verstehen Explained

The previous chapter introduced the concept of *Verstehen* as a key alternative to the biopsychosocial (BPS) model. Some readers will want more detail, though; so now our thinking caps will really be needed, as we try to deepen our understanding of the meaning of *meaning*. (This chapter is philosophical and somewhat unavoidably technical at times; it can be skipped by those already convinced of the rationale and utility of the *Verstehen* concept.)

The Rise of Science

To better understand *Verstehen*, we might begin with the major impact of science, especially Newtonian physics and Darwinian biology, on the nineteenth-century Western world (Von Wright 1971; Truzzi 1974; Makkreel 1992). These revolutions in science also affected religion, philosophy, history, and all the humanities. Newton showed that the world could be subsumed under clear physical laws that could be understood by human reason. Understanding these laws had practical benefits: physics led to engineering, science produced technology, and the industrial revolution vastly improved the life of humankind. Darwin showed that the human body and the world of nature also could be subsumed under biological laws that could be understood by human reason. The implications of his ideas provided a scientific rationale for what previously had been explained only by religion and myth.

The power of Newton and Darwin as exemplars of modern science was immense. Philosophers took note, and some of them began to feel that the methods of modern science should be applied everywhere, not just in physics and biology but also in philosophy, religion, history, and literature. At the lead of this pack was Auguste Comte, the mid-nineteenth-century French philosopher who is generally seen as the founder of the positivistic philosophy of science, as well as of modern sociology. Comte claimed that humanity had gone through prior stages of religious belief, followed by rationalist philosophy, and had finally arrived at the state of positive knowledge based on science. Science revealed the actual facts of the world, the real positive things that exist, as they are, without any distortion or error. This is the view of science that is called *positivism,* and, as Ralph Waldo Emerson put it in another context, most modern human beings are positivists in their bones. We may never have read or heard of Comte, but this interpretation of science is the one we implicitly accept in our culture. Another important figure was Thomas H. Huxley, a friend of Darwin, who argued that scientific training was key to modern education and that classic humanistic fields needed to be replaced by scientifically oriented thinking. Huxley had a famous debate with British poet Matthew Arnold about the merits of science versus the humanities, a precursor to C. P. Snow's 1959 lecture on the "two cultures."

By the late nineteenth century, science was on the offensive; religion and the traditional humanities were reeling; philosophy and academic humanists were wavering.

The Attempt to Accept Science but Reject Positivism

Here is where an interesting group of thinkers popped up. They were generally scientifically trained and thus sympathetic to science. They had often been raised in religious households, so their fathers' religion had also seeped into their bones. While they had consciously banished religious faith from their beliefs, being agnostic or atheist, they were not antireligious either. They saw that the faiths of the past could not hold, but their experience with science suggested to them that the new religion of positivism was a poor substitute.

This group was not homogenous, and most intellectual historians have not grouped them together, but they share a common aversion to positivism along with a healthy respect for science. Here we find the most uniquely American contribution to modern philosophy: pragmatism (Menand 2002). The leading figures of this way of thinking, indeed its founders, were Charles Sanders Peirce and William James. Later figures that followed in the wake of this approach were John Dewey and W. V. O. Quine. Through Quine, this attitude has had extensive influence in contemporary American philosophy, among such thinkers as Daniel Dennett and Richard Rorty. In Europe, the leading figure was Wilhelm Dilthey (sometimes called the "German William James" [Ermarth 1978]). In fact, in 1867, Dilthey and James once had dinner together at the home of a mutual friend; both were young and not yet famous, and they were impressed by each other. Dilthey later explicitly valued and approved of James's philosophical oeuvre (Ermarth 1978, p. 33). Along with Dilthey, Edmund Husserl and Franz Brentano represent late nineteenth-century European thinkers who were neither positivist nor idealist. This founding European generation of thinkers was followed by Max Weber, who in turn had a profound and direct influence on Karl Jaspers. Jaspers and Martin Heidegger (both also affected by Dilthey and Husserl) founded the philosophical school of phenomenology and existentialism.

Thus, we have an extensive intellectual gold mine on which to draw in our discussion of *Verstehen*. All these thinkers had rejected, under the impact of modern science, the verities of the past: traditional religion and idealism and old-fashioned metaphysics had no role for them; at the same time, they all also saw the flaws of positivism, the dangers of science run wild. They struggled with how to better understand science, as well as the human studies. I focus on three figures—Dilthey, Weber, and Dennett—and briefly look at Jaspers too in examining how this worldview is best applied to psychiatry and medicine.

Wilhelm Dilthey

Wilhelm Dilthey is the key figure for understanding science in late nineteenth-century Germany, as well as for appreciating how science applies to human studies (Ermarth 1978). Dilthey made the basic distinction that one cannot use the same methods for the study of human beings as one uses for the study of rocks, ions, or atoms. In other words, the methods of the natural sciences differ from the methods of the human studies (by which he meant the social sciences plus the humanities).[1] For Dilthey, this seemed obvious: "We know natural objects from without through our senses. . . . How different is the way mental life is given to us! In contrast to external perception, inner perception rests on an awareness, a lived experience (*Erlebnis*), it is immediately given. . . . We can now mark off the human studies from the natural sciences by quite clear criteria. These lie in the attitude of mind described above" (Dilthey 1974, pp. 15–16).

The distinction was thus primarily (though not completely, as described below) epistemological. The way we think, how we know, is just different when we are doing physics from when we are doing politics. This does not make politics inherently unscientific and physics inherently scientific, as the positivists would claim. It does mean that we need to appreciate to what extent, and how, scientific knowledge exists in these different domains.

In the case of natural sciences, the methods are well known: observation of empirical facts, constructions of hypotheses based on those facts, and testing of those hypotheses on new observations. This procedure could be augmented by experiment, where all factors are kept equal except one, so as to assess whether that factor has a causal effect on observed changes in the empirical world. Observation, hypothesis, and experiment, in the context of the observed external world, often with the aid of mathematical (statistical) evaluation—this is the method of natural science. As discussed previously, Dilthey termed this approach *Erklären* (to clarify), translated as "causal explanation."

In the case of the human studies, Dilthey asserted that three aspects came into play: first, the "lived experience" or *Erlebnis* of the person or persons being studied is inferred. This process occurs through empathy (*Einfuhling;* though Dilthey preferred the terms "reliving" or "transposition" of oneself into the place of the other). This first-person lived experience is then augmented by the "expressions" of the other person—what she says verbally and how she acts nonverbally, perhaps even through direct dialogues with that person. This second step is then followed by the full cognitive act of understanding, the attempt to put it all together into some kind of meaning that makes sense of the behavior being observed, or of the human topic being studied ("synthetic meaning"; Ermarth 1978; Makkreel 1992).[2] As defined in the last chapter, there is a triad to *Verstehen*: *Erlebnis*, expressions, and synthetic meaning.

The Verstehen *Debate*

Exactly what Dilthey meant by the concept of *Verstehen* has been the source of considerable debate for most of the nearly a hundred years since his death. This debate has lingered partly because most of Dilthey's writings have remained unpublished even in German, not to mention mostly untranslated into other tongues; they were released in his collected works in dribs and drabs (his collected writings now number more than seventeen volumes, and other volumes continue to come out). This gradual discovery of Dilthey's ideas contrasts with the fact that in his own lifetime he only published three books (*Introduction to the Human Sciences, Poetics,* and *Life of Schleiermacher*), and thus his contemporaries judged him mainly on these limited published sources. Much has been made of Dilthey's reticence to publish in his later decades. Perhaps, as chair of philosophy in Berlin, holding the seat previously occupied by the great Hegel, Dilthey felt little academic pressure to publish; perhaps, as many hold, he was too much of a perfectionist, not yet feeling his work was clear or complete enough to be brought to published light; perhaps, as some of his detractors say, he was too murky in his thought and unable to clarify it enough to publish. Whatever is the case, the interpretations of his works have suffered from their published incompleteness.

Like some other great thinkers, Dilthey lived long enough to produce works that allow for early, middle, and late monikers. One cannot say with such figures that the later writings are the best, or necessarily the final, versions of their thought, though many tend to assume so. In some sense, there is no single correct answer; it is our judgment as interpreters that matters.

This background is relevant to appreciating what Dilthey meant by *Verstehen,* because he meant different things by it in different phases of his life. In his early years, he emphasized its psychological components, such as empathy and re-experiencing. He even held that psychology as a discipline was the central field of the human studies. He was roundly criticized for this view by others, particularly Heidelberg philosopher Heinrich Rickert, who wanted the human studies to be reflected more in the social sciences, like sociology, rather than the arts and the humanities (which for him included psychology). (Rickert thus preferred the term "cultural sciences" or *Kulturwissenschaften,* rather than *Geisteswissenschaften.*) Dilthey never came to agree with Rickert's rejection of psychology, but Dilthey did, over time, lessen his emphasis on psychology as the central discipline of the human studies and put less and less emphasis on psychological concepts as part of his explication of *Verstehen.* Instead, he increased emphasis on the creation of meaning. One reason for Dilthey's evolution away from psychology was his unhappiness with the state of the discipline in the late 1890s. Influenced by Wilhelm Wundt (a mentor to Emil Kraepelin), psychology was experimental and objective; Dilthey was more interested in a psychology that was descriptive and subjective. Hence, in his later years, his thought began to converge with the ideas of Edmund Husserl, the founder of the field of phenomenology; Husserl later acknowledged that Dilthey was avant-garde in his wish for a phenomenological (subjective, internally oriented) psychology, as opposed to Wundt's purely external, behavioristic, experimental psychology (Makkreel 1992).

Meaning versus Empathy

The early Dilthey is sometimes labeled "psychologistic" and the later Dilthey "hermeneutic" (Makkreel 1991). Differing interpretations sometimes cull from different eras in Dilthey's work. Thus, one commentator emphasizes the psychologistic Dilthey's view of *Verstehen*: "It is possible . . . to say in a few words what distinguishes the human world from the world of nature sufficiently to require and justify a distinctive method of research. Human beings talk, while the rest of nature is mute, or, at least, as is the case with higher animals, inarticulate. So what we learn about human beings is based on communications from beings like us, not just on observation of objects and events" (Rickman 1988).

In contrast, philosopher Rudolph Makkreel, a leading expert on Dilthey, emphasizes the later hermeneutic thinker:

> Dilthey distinguishes between abstraction and analysis. Both start with a whole, but abstraction "singles out one fact and disregards the others, whereas [analysis] seeks to apprehend the majority of the facts that make up the factors of a complex whole.". . . Abstraction is associated especially with explanations of the natural sciences. Analysis in the sense of considering parts on the basis of the whole can be said to engender the understanding which Dilthey claims is "central" to the human sciences. To understand a person is to localize partial states in relation to "the structure of the whole of psychic life." In understanding, "structure is everything! And we cannot avoid the circle: From the complex of data given to me I generate the total nexus of a psychic structure in which I interpret the particular on the basis of the whole, and the whole on the basis of the particular." (Makkreel 1992)

Although the term *analysis* is confusing to modern readers in this setting, what Dilthey is emphasizing here is that *Erklären* focuses on abstraction from reality (such as creating general laws from empirical facts), while *Verstehen* focuses on holistic interpretation, understanding the parts on the basis of the whole. (For modern readers, the term *analysis* best relates to *Erklären*-based assessment of separate facts and their relation to general laws, while the term *synthesis* is applied to Dilthey's concept of *Verstehen*-based attention to holistic phenomena.)

Dilthey is often seen as prefiguring the later hermeneutic tradition in philosophy, partly based on his later emphasis on the centrality of meaning for *Verstehen*.

Even so, Dilthey always emphasized the validity of the natural sciences and of their method (*Erklären*), in their own sphere. He also held that *Erklären* was even useful in the human studies. Thus, he was not trying to privilege *Verstehen* over *Erklären*, or vice versa; he was trying to give each its due. In contrast, some later hermeneutic and postmodern philosophers, like Jürgen Habermas, are critical of Dilthey for not seeing *Verstehen* as the be-all and end-all of knowledge. Others, as Makkreel notes, view Dilthey as too much of a protopositivist, because he accepted the methods of nineteenth-century positivist natural science within their own fields. Of course, much work has been done in philosophy of science showing that, even within the natural and physical sciences, *Erklären* is not as simple a method as it may have seemed in the nineteenth century. For instance, Makkreel describes how quantum physics has removed the connection of simple causality to physical explanation. In a sense, *Verstehen,* and not only *Erklären,* is at work in our understanding of physics. Makkreel explains how the work of some later philosophers, like Ernst Cassirer, took into account this evolution of physics, allowing for more clarity about *Erklären* and *Verstehen* than Dilthey might have been able to achieve, given the state of science in his era (Makkreel 1992).

Verstehen, then, to return to our theme, involves psychological components (as emphasized by the early Dilthey) and hermeneutic components (as emphasized by the later Dilthey). At one level, Dilthey's contribution was about clarifying what we mean by science and taking it beyond positivism. For Dilthey, science is not just *Erklären.* It is the systematic use of *Verstehen* and *Erklären,* emphasizing one or the other more in the natural versus human studies (also see glossary).

A Line and a Circle

A metaphor may help us clarify the relation of *Erklären* and *Verstehen,* especially as it was developed in the later Dilthey. Many have used the metaphor of a circle, as did Dilthey, to describe hermeneutic knowledge. This is often related to the concept that there is no beginning and no end to a circle; one enters it at whatever point. Further, every part of the circle is understood only in relation to the circle as a whole, and there is no specific direction of causality: the parts are needed to understand the whole, and vice versa. In contrast, one can think of *Erklären* as a straight line: one event causes another, and each event is independent of another. The general law that describes this causality derives, but is separate from, the empirical events (in place of *event,* one can also use the term *fact* or *phenomenon*). This linear causal type of explanation is what Dilthey had in mind with the concept of *Erklären.* Obviously, explanation in the physical and natural sciences is

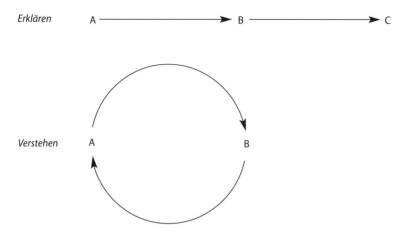

Figure 2. Erklären and *Verstehen:* A line versus a circle

more complex: nonlinear concepts now exist, along with complex notions such as parallel-processing and chaos theory. But many scientists (especially those only partly trained in science, such as doctors) tend to think about science in a serial, linear, causal way. To the extent that this kind of explanation is still relevant to the natural sciences, it is what Dilthey meant by the concept of *Erklären* (see Figure 2).

Erklären involves one event or fact (A, B, C) causing another in a serial manner. *Verstehen* involves understanding events or facts as parts related to a whole and understanding the whole as constituted by those parts. No specific direction of causality exists (the hermeneutic circle).

Knowing versus Being

The above discussion sheds light also on the question of whether *Verstehen* and *Erklären* are primarily methods of knowledge (i.e., epistemological methods only). Many have thought about it in this manner (Slavney and McHugh 1987), and one can see that this view reflects the later Dilthey in particular. Others, who focus on Dilthey's discussions of psychology, feel differently: One commentator writes (using "Understanding" to mean *Verstehen*):

> Understanding is not a method. . . . We should talk of a method based on, and aiming at, understanding, rather than the method of understanding. . . . Understanding is not an activity at all, not something we do, but something we accomplish . . . [It is] not a method, but a cognitive process. A cross-reference to observation [*Erklären*] and its relation to the scientific method may clarify this point.

Observation is crucial in, let us say, physics or astronomy . . . but observation is not a method. It is part of everyday life, and we may engage in it absentmindedly or with concentrated attention. . . . It is best described as a cognitive process that, employed systematically and combined with other processes, can become part of a method, which by contrast may be defined as a systematic combination of cognitive processes. (Rickman 1988)

An alternative view is to emphasize that *Erklären* and *Verstehen* are cognitive categories, and thus epistemological in part, though not completely. As Makkreel puts it, they are two ways of making cognitive sense of the world, but *Verstehen*, for Dilthey, is not a purely intellectual or rational process; it also involves the will and emotions—all of what constitutes the mind (Makkreel 1992):

The contrast between understanding and explanation has proven difficult to characterize; it is certainly not reducible to the simple form of immediate versus mediate knowledge so often suggested. When Dilthey writes in the *Ideen* that "We explain through purely intellectual processes, but we understand through the cooperation of all our psychic powers (*Gemütskräfte*) . . . ," it is apparent that intellectual operations are not excluded from the process of understanding. . . . In the *Ideen,* Dilthey was especially concerned with understanding as it applied to psychology. Broadly, it could be said that explanation involves subsuming the particular data or elements that can be abstracted from our experience to general laws, whereas understanding is more concerned with focusing on the concrete contents of individual processes of experience to consider how they function as part of a larger continuum. (Makkreel 1992)

In his writings on history, as opposed to psychology, Dilthey describes holistic thinking in *Verstehen,* but he stresses more the creation of meaning. Makkreel emphasizes the epistemological conditions that differentiate the natural sciences from the human studies; the former begin with hypotheses based on external observations and with attempts to explain those observations based on those hypotheses. Through a self-correcting process, those hypotheses lead to general laws, which are the ultimate result of *Erklären*. In contrast, the human studies begin with "lived experience," actual mental states and expressions and activities of human beings. This lived experience is not hypothetical, but real, and its explanation does not involve abstraction of hypotheses and creation of general laws but rather apprehending the meaning of the experience as a whole. Makkreel puts it thus:

Hypotheses can, to be sure, have as subordinate role in the *Geisteswissenschaften*, but only to the extent that we may want to fit in, and relate, isolated details of meaning. The *Naturwissenschaften*, on the other hand, do not start with a lived continuum, so that connections between purely physical states or atomic particles are merely hypothetical. On the basis of this difference in the epistemological conditions of the *Wissenschaften*, we can uncover a division within classification as such. In the *Geisteswissenschaften*, where connectedness is primary, the rationale for classification must lie in articulating appropriate divisions. Thus we find that the hermeneutic circle converges on the typical parts of a whole. In the *Naturwissenschaften*, the main goal of classification would be that of overcoming any initial discontinuities and discovering similarities and hypothetical connections. Thus it is that natural description leads to inductive uniformities whereby ever more particulars can be subsumed under universal laws. (Makkreel 1992)

Psychology versus History

The early Dilthey emphasized psychology as the central discipline of the human studies; the later Dilthey turned to history, not as the central discipline, but as the most *complex* discipline, among the human studies (Makkreel 1992). The emphasis on history is key for understanding Dilthey, for an unfinished project—perhaps the central project of his life's work—was his *Critique of Historical Reason*. The title echoes Immanuel Kant, and Makkreel feels that Dilthey's work can be best interpreted as an attempt to extend Kant's *Critique of Pure Reason*, which applied to physics and the natural sciences, to the human studies (Makkreel 1992; Ermarth 1978). In other words, Kant's philosophical contribution was limited to the natural sciences, although Kant saw it as applicable to all knowledge. Hegel first noted that human history might stand outside the Kantian paradigm, and Dilthey was trying to take that Hegelian insight further and to work out the actual logic of history (and all the human studies), so as to complement Kant's insights into the logic of the physical sciences (Makkreel 1992).

Another way of putting this, to highlight how all of these thinkers were reacting and responding to the evolution of science, might be as follows: Kant was faced with Newton. He asked himself: If the physical world is as Newton has shown it to be, what does that mean for humanity? How does it affect our understanding of how we know, and of what we know, and even of what we believe, or how we should behave? Dilthey was faced with Darwin. He asked himself: If the natural world is as Darwin has shown it to be, what does that mean for humanity?

And today, we are still faced with Newton and Darwin, and we might add now

Freud and Einstein and DNA. Those aspects of science should be directing us back to better understanding Kant and Dilthey, so as to move forward from where they took us.

Dilthey's Method-Based Philosophy

A final point: the distinction between *Erklären* and *Verstehen* does not necessarily mean that there are two worlds that differ from each other, where these two perspectives need to be used completely in separation from each other.[3] Some critics of Dilthey ascribe this view to him (e.g., his contemporary Rickert; Oakes 1988), but Dilthey was not making the claim of two different realms of being (an ontological distinction), nor even a claim about two completely different ways of knowing (an epistemological claim). Nor did he subscribe to Rickert's view, also promoted by Max Weber (see below), that the distinction between *Erklären* and *Verstehen* had to do mainly with our interests or our values (a pragmatic or axiological distinction). Dilthey did emphasize aspects of these perspectives, particularly pragmatic and epistemological rationales, but he did not claim that one criterion of demarcation clearly sufficed. He cared about the matter and spent much of his work trying to clarify the rationale for distinguishing *Erklären* and *Verstehen,* but he refused to simplify it. For him, these were two cognitive approaches to understanding the world, one of which had to do with nature and the other with human beings; they could and should both be used in all aspects of knowledge, but they had different strengths and limitations, applying best differentially in the separate arenas of natural science and the human studies.

Criticisms of Verstehen

These are the meanings of *Verstehen,* as initiated by Dilthey, and they have faced a number of criticisms. The most common critique identifies *Verstehen* with just the first step: *Erlebnis;* the claim is that empathy is just touchy-feely; it is clearly not science, because it is almost impossible to generalize, teach, or describe. Beyond the fact that these assumptions are not true (there is a wonderful psychiatric literature on how to learn and practice empathy; Havens 1986; Marguelis 1989), this critique mistakes all of *Verstehen* with the first step of it.

Not appreciating the above fact, others have been skeptical about *Verstehen* because they see it as simply empathic acceptance of the behavior of others (Abel 1974). This empathy does not add to human knowledge, in this view. But Dilthey saw *Verstehen* as a way to better understand (*Besser Verstehen;* Ermarth 1978) a human event than it was understood by those involved in those events: by examining all the facts and evidence surrounding Napoleon's invasion of Russia, we might be able to construct a *Verstehen* theory that would better understand why he invaded Russia than Napoleon himself could have known or explained the day that he signed the marching orders. It is not simply a matter of pure empathy, of trying to appreciate what he thought; it is about finding out the truth about why he did what he did.

Another critique is that *Verstehen* is not science because it is not general; it is all about individual human beings, and our relation to individuals can never reach the level of science, which requires general descriptions and laws (Nagel 1953; Hempel 1965). This view of *Verstehen* makes it the method of *idiographic* knowledge, or knowledge of individuals in their uniqueness, as opposed to *nomologic* knowledge, or knowledge of groups in their shared general properties. Heinrich Rickert, a contemporary of Dilthey, held this view, but Dilthey directly rejected it (Ermarth 1978). For Dilthey, the final step of knowledge in the human studies, *Verstehen,* involved putting together *Erlebnis* and verbal and nonverbal expressions to form some kind of general judgments about the nature of the human topic being studied. This general judgment could apply to large groups, societies, nations, and races; it did not have to be limited to unique individuals.

Another critique is that lived experience and expressions involve inferences that are not scientific, but simply common sense, and are thus markedly fallible (Abel 1974). Dilthey himself might have inadvertently encouraged this dismissive attitude by emphasizing how *Verstehen* begins by using commonsense interpretations. If you see a thin man, with dry lips, panting in front of a hot roast beef sandwich and then eating it with ravaging gusto, you likely would be justified in making the commonsense inference that he was hungry. Dilthey used this kind of example to try to show that *Verstehen* was not something mysterious but rather a method of knowing that we use all the time. His critics look at this kind of example, though, and contrast it with the pretty colors and complex computerized equations that go into an MRI image, and they see the former as nonscience and the latter as science. Einstein's dictum that science is nothing but refined everyday thinking (Einstein 1950) shows us what Dilthey meant. *Verstehen* is science, so is *Erklären;* the former in a certain field, the latter in another (Wiggins and Schwartz 1991). Max Weber showed how this commonsense *Verstehen* could be further refined so that it became more useful as a tool of scientific knowledge—as "ideal types" (see below).

A final critique might be that all human knowledge is one; the distinction into two types is unjustified (Martin 1969; Wilson 1998). In fact, Dilthey did not argue that these were two separate kinds of knowledge, each unique to its own field.

Rather, Dilthey's view was that these two ways of knowing, these two approaches to life and knowledge, are not mutually incompatible. They are matters of emphasis. In the natural sciences, we mostly use *Erklären*, but we also somewhat use *Verstehen*. In the human studies, we mostly use *Verstehen*, but we also somewhat use *Erklären*. It is not a matter of all-or-none; these are not airtight compartments. Rather, Dilthey's concern was that, in a world of positivism run amuck, the case had to be made for some role of *Verstehen* in human knowledge (Ermarth 1978). How do we use *Verstehen* in the natural sciences? Weber's work provides an example, but I'll use a more general example (later developed by Dennett [1995])—the concept of evolution. Evolution, at least in some biological theories, involves teleology: there is a purpose to it—namely survival of the specific animal and its genes. How do we know that survival is the goal of evolution? We don't. We infer this purpose, we posit it, out of thin air. Why? Because it makes sense of a whole host of data, as Darwin marshaled in his classic work. By positing the goal of survival, we can explain many facts regarding the observed distribution of species in nature. So we have used *Verstehen*, the postulate of a purpose, to propose the law of evolution, which we derived from and tested further based on empirical observation.

Conversely, how do we use *Erklären* in the human studies? Just because *Verstehen* is needed, one cannot conclude that it is all that is needed. If I want to understand why Napoleon invaded Russia, it does not hurt, and may even help, my overall interpretative effort if I know exactly how many soldiers were in Napoleon's army, how much money he had in his banks, how many soldiers were in the Russian army, the state of the Russian purse, the length and severity of the Russian winter, and so on. These are all facts and figures—numbers—that are just as quantified as the level of sodium in the blood. They can be statistically analyzed. Thus, *Erklären* can be, and should be, used in the human studies; Dilthey's point was that it does not exhaust human phenomena.

Max Weber

We now come to Max Weber, a founder of sociology. He was influenced by both Dilthey and Rickert (Oakes 1988) and thus more directly describes *Verstehen* as related to understanding individual behavior (as did Rickert, but not Dilthey); hence the concept of *Verstehen* has been pilloried in the sociological literature as being purely a matter of individual psychology (God forbid; Truzzi 1974). We have seen that this need not be the case, and I focus instead on Weber's contribution regarding the "ideal type" concept, which I see as the systematization and refinement of Dilthey's *Verstehen* (the result of the triad of lived experience, expressions, and synthetic meaning). Weber's ideal type is Dilthey's *Verstehen* honed and shined so as to apply to sociology (Tucker 1965). Weber saw it as the way to get past all the individual, unique (idiographic) morass of facts that occur in human phenomena. This infinite number of unique varieties of human experience are abstracted by the sociologist into basic types (here too Dilthey had prefigured the importance of the cognitive construct of *types;* he applied it to history). These ideal types do not in fact exist in nature, but they provide an abstraction from the messy natural world to a more clear and understandable abstract theory. This theory, the product of *Verstehen,* can then be re-examined and tested in the real world of observed human social phenomena (McIntosh 1977).

Here is how Weber puts it, with my commentary in brackets:

> To understand . . . means interpretive understanding of a.) concrete individual cases, as for example in historical analysis [here he refers to Rickert's idiographic knowledge]; b.) average cases, that is approximate estimates [i.e., *Erklären*] . . . ; or c.) a pure type of a frequently occurring scientifically formulated construct [ideal types]. Such ideally typical constructs are, for example, the concepts and axioms of pure economic theory. They show how a given type of human behavior would occur, on a strictly rational basis, unaffected by errors or emotional factors, and if, further, it were directed to a single goal. Actual behavior takes this course only rarely [e.g., on the stock exchange] and then only approximately so as to correspond to the ideal type. (Weber 1974, pp. 25–26)

Weber's extensive corpus makes difficult reading when it comes to methodology, however, and thus his key concept of ideal types is mostly presented in concrete examples in his work, rather than theoretical discussion. His successors debated the idea more conceptually, making for an extensive sociological literature pro and con. His direct disciple, Karl Jaspers, defines ideal types thus:

> Reality is an infinite weaving of the meaningful and the meaningless. In order to seize it, constructed concepts are necessary which, developed in themselves as meaningfully consistent, serve only as standards for reality, to see how far it conforms to those concepts. Weber calls these constructed concepts ideal types. To him, they are the perceptive-technical means of approaching reality, not reality itself. They are . . . meaningful concepts by which reality is measured, in so far as it corresponds to them, in order to precisely comprehend it and to bring out

clearly as a fact the element that does not conform to them. They are not the aim of knowledge, not the laws of what has happened, but a means to gain the clearest awareness of the specific characteristics of human reality at the present time. The wealth of Weberian insights rests on the construction of such ideal types, demonstrated as fruitful for the concrete knowledge of the real. (Jaspers 1989, pp. 87–88)

Verstehen is followed by *Erklären* in Weber's sociology. He uses both, just as Dilthey supported. Neither thinker argued, contrary to modern critics, that history or sociology should consist of nothing but *Verstehen,* without any attention to or interest in empirical facts or statistical methods. Rather, both methods needed to be used in appropriate ways. By ignoring *Verstehen* and trying to impose empirical methods where they do not apply or ignoring human phenomena that cannot be easily measured directly, the positivistic approach to history and sociology leads to a pallid history that fails to instruct and a sickly sociology that fails to enlighten. In contrast, Weber's work on the relation of Calvinism to the rise of capitalism, his contributions on the importance of bureaucracy in modern society, and his insights into the role of charisma in leadership—to mention a few of his ideas—have stood the test of time (Gerth and Mills 1948).

Weber's ideal type concept may also be useful for understanding psychiatric diagnosis, as Jaspers claimed. For instance, Michael Schwartz and Osbourne Wiggins describe how many current controversies about the various editions of the *Diagnostic and Statistical Manual of Mental Disorders* are based on positivistic assumptions, whereas ideal type methods may be more fruitful (Schwartz and Wiggins 1986, 1987).

Daniel Dennett's Intentional Stance

Finally, I highlight one contemporary thinker whose ideas also point out the importance of this *Erklären-Verstehen* distinction, one who would not typically be identified with the nonscientific assumptions that are often attributed to the *Verstehen* school (a critique that is false, as I have shown, because *Verstehen* is put forward not as an alternative to science per se, but as an alternative to positivistic science). That thinker is Daniel Dennett, a scientifically minded philosopher of mind, a strict materialist and proponent of Darwinism in philosophy and religion. Dennett posits three ways in which we have knowledge about ourselves and the world, which he calls *stances* (Dennett 1991): The first is the *intentional stance,* whereby we infer reasons based on the assumption of rationality in others and through inference of their internal mental states. If someone appears hungry, sees food, and eats it, we draw the rational inference that the reason this person ate that food was because he was hungry. This is the world of commonsense thinking, which Dennett calls *folk psychology.* The second approach is the *design stance;* this is where we judge something based on what it appears designed to do. For artificial things, like a table, we make the judgment that the creator of the table had designed it so that it would be used to hold things. For natural things, like species, we have come upon a theory of natural selection to explain the purpose or design behind the observed distribution of species. A third and final approach is the *physical stance,* the idea that we best explain some things by understanding what they are made of in physical terms. Thus, if I want to know the nature of water, it might be useful to find out that it is composed of two hydrogen and one oxygen atom. Dennett uses these concepts to explain the complexity of understanding human consciousness. The simple application of any one stance seems wrong: for instance, a purely materialist identification of every mental state with a brain state would simply be application of the physical stance as the sole solution to the problem of consciousness. For many reasons, this does not work. Others apply concepts from folk psychology, without any role for the brain; this attitude (which comprises much academic philosophy) also fails to explain consciousness. Still others take a pure design stance, as in artificial intelligence. Dennett himself has used the design stance when applying Darwinian approaches to consciousness.

The larger points are that no single stance is sufficient for all knowledge, that each stance has its own strengths and limitations, and that part of the work of science (and philosophy) is to determine which stance applies best and in which settings to promote valid knowledge. This approach is consistent with the method-based philosophy found at the heart of Dilthey, William James, Charles Sanders Peirce, and the main body of pragmatic philosophy, as well as in Jaspers, most notably, among the phenomenological school.

Dennett (1991) also uses the term *heterophenomenology* (the phenomenology of others than oneself) to denote how we obtain information about the mental states of others and ourselves, in the course of engaging in the scientific work of psychology and the social sciences, as well as in our daily living. This heterophenomenology reflects the use of the intentional stance in part but also much of what Dilthey termed *Verstehen,* especially the second part of the *Verstehen* triad—careful attention to people's verbal and nonverbal expressions. Subjectivity, and the commonly used language of first-person experience, according to Dennett, is another way of saying that we are engaging in heterophenomenology.

If one wishes to trace historical similarities, one might see the intentional stance as similar to what Dilthey meant by *Verstehen* (though not all of it), as is the design stance. The physical stance seems to correspond to *Erklären*, as does part of the design stance (e.g., the observational evidence underlying natural selection or the mathematical calculations of artificial intelligence).

The insights of *Verstehen* seem to have relevance to modern philosophy of mind.

The End of Positivism

In sum, there is a role for a kind of knowledge that is not purely about numbers, empirical observations, experiment, and statistics. Not all knowledge is purely empirical; science is not equivalent to positivism; Comte was not the last word.

All this seems obvious once it is explained; but it needs explaining, because today we live with positivism as an unspoken assumption, transmitted to us, in the Western world, along with the placental fluid that passed around us *in utero*.

Modern philosophy of science has long bypassed positivism; all data need to be interpreted; all observations are theory-laden; hypothesis is as key to science as observation or experiment. These are basic maxims about modern science, nonpositivistic interpretations, commonly attributed to names like Thomas Kuhn and Karl Popper, but long ago similarly expressed by Dilthey, Weber, James, and Peirce. The German tradition in particular tried to explain this reality with the concept of *Verstehen*, but years of positivistic critique, especially in sociology, have put *Verstehen* in disrepute.

Perhaps we should resuscitate the concept of *Verstehen*, especially in psychiatry, to better appreciate what science means, what kind of knowledge we possess, and how best to apply these two basic methods of *Erklären* and *Verstehen* in advancing knowledge in this discipline that sits smack dab in the middle between the natural sciences and the human studies.

CHAPTER SIXTEEN

The Beginning of a Solution

Method-Based Psychiatry

In 1965, psychiatrist Roy Grinker, whom readers should now appreciate as the founder of eclectic psychiatry, related a parable that he hoped would explain why psychiatry needed to be eclectic; he called it "the land of human behavior" (Grinker 1965). One might call this story "Grinker's Dream," because though so true in many respects, it ended in a fantasy, one that became a reality, and is now a nightmare (Grinker 1965):

> A certain foreign country in a far away continent somewhere in the cosmos is called the Land of Human Behavior. In it there are large and small areas fenced off for the growth and development of special crops by methods called *disciplines*. Most of these fences have variable-sized openings through which neighbors from near and far pass in various directions. These communicate with the local residents and exchange advice with them about how to grow a variety of crops known as *sciences*. Through communication in understandable language an exchange of *information* is effected.
>
> Some people produce little but carefully study the processes of growth and development in their own and other fields. They are helpful to the entire population but are not appreciated because they seem to have no prediction for one method or one crop.

In some areas the inhabitants own many horses and they periodically ride madly in all directions, tarrying briefly in the communities called family, society and nations where they at talk at length about mankind in general, prevention of war and social change. They are serious and well motivated but they neglect their own fields and grow little. These people are called *planners* and they need not toil in the field because they are well supported by their rich Uncle Sam.

Some areas are almost completely fenced off, and the inhabitants compulsively tend to strengthen their fences at the slightest criticism from their neighbors. When people from other areas attempt to visit them they become unhappy and build another fence inside those already existing, thereby restricting themselves more and more as they exclude the unanalyzed strangers. They teach their rituals to their young in an old-fashioned way, and those pupils who do not learn or remember properly are vigorously expelled. These inhabitants of *Freudiana* plant only a few seeds at a time but they nourish them carefully for years, and if the results turn out to be somewhat peculiar, they start with different seeds but use exactly the same procedure as before. These people communicate only in dyads, and because of many dialects the can hardly understand each other when they talk about inferences and intuition.

Closely related to the Freudians are people who live at the opposite part of the country. These are called cosmologists, humanist, religionists and *existentialists;* they barely talk to the others, and when they speak their language is largely unintelligible. They grow peculiar and exotic-looking crops which apparently have no use and about which they are sentimental. They abhor scientism and are bitter about facing facts.

Somewhere in the center of the country is a small group of individuals who have migrated from all parts, thus representing many fields and various kinds of farmers and riders. These people are engaged in formulating general rules applicable to all functions carried on in the Land of Human Behavior. They are called *unifiers* or systems-theorists; they are accepted by few and their influence is minimal. Yet they can endure the studied neglect of most an even the name-calling by the isolates, for they have faith in science and the scientific method. (italics in original)

Kety's Parable

Grinker's "unifiers"—the eclectic thinkers—formulated the biopsychosocial (BPS) model on the outlines he constructed. Psychiatry accepted this new way of thinking a generation ago. Today, their influence is hardly minimal; in fact, they now represent the power structure of psychiatry. Though this eclecticism is to be preferred to the dogmas of the past, it has not led to a clarifying unified theory of psychiatry.

We are now faced with a hodge-podge of facts and theories, and we need more than Grinker envisioned in his parable. A few years earlier, psychiatric researcher Seymour Kety proposed another parable, *The True Nature of a Book* (Kety 1960),[1] similar to Grinker's story, but perhaps more profound. In Kety's tale, a book fell into a planet, and the inhabitants there convened their researchers and thinkers to try to read it, because it was written in unintelligible script. The biologists assessed the cellular structure of its pages, the chemists its atomic content, the physiologists the ruffling of its spine, the psychologists the number of occurrences of certain word-markings, and finally they turned the whole matter over to the molecular biologists, those with the shiniest and newest instruments. With the motto: "No twisted book without a twisted molecule," the molecular biologists indeed discovered that the book was composed of a twisted molecule: cellulose. Yet everyone remained in the dark as to the meaning of its markings. At last, the psychoanalysts were called; they sat down with others and asked them to describe whatever came to mind as they read the book.

Kety's parable is more pessimistic and accurate than is Grinker's fantasy. No one of those investigators truly understood the book; no one had a monopoly of knowledge; and there was no way to put together all of their disparate perspectives to obtain a "holistic" or "integrated" knowledge of the book.[2]

Perhaps there is only one valid method of knowing what is in the book: read it. All the other methods might teach us something, but not much, until that planet develops the language skills to be able to translate and read the book.

This is a method-based psychiatry that is neither eclectic nor dogmatic, an approach in which no single method applies to all aspects of psychiatry, but also in which one method is better than a mix of many. The task of scientific research and conceptual thinking is to identify those methods that are best appropriate for their specific goals or purposes.[3]

A Medical Democracy

There is an alternative to both eclecticism and dogmatism; following Havens, I have called it *pluralism,* which may not be the best term, because most Americans equate it with eclecticism (see glossary). Perhaps a better phrase would be *method-*

based psychiatry (see previous chapter), in analogy and contrast to evidence-based medicine.

Let the reader identify pluralism with method-based psychiatry, then, and the following political analogies may be helpful:

If eclecticism is anarchy and dogmatism tyranny, then pluralism is democracy. With eclecticism, anything goes: we live in a Nietzschean world where all is permitted, and nothing is punished. In a lawless world, injustice becomes the norm. The hard hand of tyranny may seem appealing, but the peace of the slave is the grave of scientific progress. Any ideology provides reasons to refuse certain ideas, but more of than not, such refusals are peremptory and false.

We want to live in a world of medical democracy, a place where psychiatrists and psychologists and social workers can say: "This is right, and that is wrong, and this is why." And they can do so without unjustly accepting a false theory or equally unjustly rejecting a true one.

Just as in a political democracy, our medical democracy will have its flaws. Different ideas will be free to battle with each other in the marketplace of ideas, as John Stuart Mill (2008) famously claimed; confusion will ensue, uncertainty will be common. This is not a world for those who prefer the security of tradition: all ideas are up for grabs, and, we expect, through scientific communication and competition, the best of them will prove fruitful, replicate, and take hold. The worse will fall away.

Some will complain: there are too many questions; this is too much uncertainty. One can only reply (as Winston Churchill did about democracy) that method-based psychiatry is the worst system, except for all the rest.

Karl Jaspers: The Third Great Germanic Psychiatrist

Give me some examples, says the reader. I have read sixteen chapters; you have completely disenchanted me from every possible theory in psychiatry; now what should I do?

Such impatience is to be applauded, but only if we remember that the truth is not something for me, the author, to give to you, the reader. It is something (as Karl Jaspers was fond of saying) *on the way.* Keep reading: the truth is with you, on your right and on your left. The last chapter began the process of revealing a key alternative.

Let's discuss the method-based approach to psychiatry, beginning in the beginning, with the founder of the whole idea: Karl Jaspers. He is the grand old man of method-based psychiatry; some might see me and others like me who are fond of him as engaging in our own kind of hero-worship, perhaps even dogmatism. We decry Freud, the old ideologue; we admonish Kraepelin, the dry reductionist: Give us Jaspers, the catholic thinker, the old-school Enlightenment figure.

At a personal level, all three Germanic thinkers are to be admired: Freud the courageous innovator, Kraepelin the creative scientist, and Jaspers the wise thinker. Personally, I plead guilty to hero-worship of all three; but, intellectually, I deny worship of any of them. Such was Jaspers's teaching: Do not worship me, or anyone else, he taught—the truth is not to be found in one place, but dispersed in all places; not just in the august halls of our old universities, but next to the old lady at the bakery, and the child on the playground, and by the mosquito in the swamp, and the flower in the valley. The truth is prosaic, not pompous: Seek it everywhere. But it is not the same in all places; this is where Jaspers's views on science come in.

In thinking about the nature of psychiatry, Jaspers discerned that there was no way to make progress by simply pitting biological approaches (as advanced by Wilhelm Griesinger and Kraepelin) against psychological approaches (as advanced by Freud and Pierre Janet). Neither was fully right, neither fully wrong; their critiques of each other were apt. Jaspers was convinced by everyone and by no one. What was he to do?

Freud versus Kraepelin

To solve the puzzle of what to do when all systems seemed partially right and partially wrong, Jaspers invented method-based psychiatry: He realized that the reason each side seemed convincing was because it directed its vision toward certain aspects of reality that the other side missed. Each school of thought did so by using a different method: Methodology determined their strengths and their weaknesses. Their theories rose and fell with their methods.

This is just science (see glossary). If I take a microscope and look at your skin, I'll see a bunch of cells; if I use an electron microscope, I'll see specific layers of cells. If I take a biopsy and centrifuge in special test tubes, I'll determine its composition based on different kinds of proteins and fatty acids. If I look at your skin with my eyes, at a meter's distance, I'll behold its smoothness and freedom from blemish. It's the same skin, looked at with different methods. What's the right way? It depends on what I want to do, my pragmatic purpose in caring to look at your skin. Is one method inherently better than the rest? Yes: if I care to see how pretty you are, looking with my eyes is best; if I want to see if you have skin cancer, look-ing with my microscope is better.

The biopsychosocial model implies that, to appreciate your skin, I need to understand it at all those levels. What Jaspers argued—what I suggest—is that this is not the case. For oncology purposes, my aesthetic feeling about the allure of the skin on your lips does not matter. For erotic purposes, the G protein composition of your subdermal layer disinterests me.

What was Freud doing? He was treating community patients with neuroses. And Kraepelin? Hospitalized patients with psychoses. How could they possibly reach the same conclusions? Freud found he needed to use the method of free as-sociation, listening to his patients without theory (at least initially) and looking for hidden meanings in apparently unimportant words. Kraepelin concluded that he needed to look at, rather than listen to, to his patients: Observing their behavior, moods, and actions, he noted salient facts, recorded them on note cards, and sat back to see what happened to them. How long did they stay in hospital? How long did they stay away? How frequently did they come back? For Freud, the uncon-scious was the royal road to knowledge; for Kraepelin, diagnosis was prognosis: the course of the patient's symptoms would tell you what his illness was.

They were both right; they were both wrong; for they were only partially right and universally wrong.

Freud was right for the people he treated and for his purposes, and Kraepelin for his. What Jaspers discerned—something which the other two men, for all their genius, failed to grasp—is that it is the nature of science that all knowledge is par-tial: no scientific theory can have validity outside of its chosen scope.

This is the method-based intuition, one which lies at the heart of any notion of science: *our methods determine our results.* Jaspers called it methodological con-sciousness: we need to be aware of what methods we use, their strengths and lim-itations, and why we use them.

As opposed to eclecticism, there *is* a right answer: We do not live in a postmod-ernist world where everything is about my culture versus yours, about power and prestige and wealth. All that is relevant, but it is not everything: there actually is a truth, and a fact of the matter. If that were not the case, then, as postmodernist physicians, we should all be immune from malpractice, and we should all abandon forthwith any practice of medicine or clinical health care, because we are messing with people's lives, and why should we do so if it is all about power, without any right or wrong answers?

What is the right answer? It is the job of scientific work to determine what the right answer is by determining what the right question is. The question is not "What is the right theory?" but "What is the right method?" Kraepelin's method would not work for Freud's patients, neither would Freud's method for Kraepelin's patients. Different methods had been devised, correctly, for different settings, conditions, and purposes.

Verstehen and Method-Based Psychiatry

Another way of looking at Jaspers's insight is that he applied *Verstehen* to psychiatry. This occurred most directly in his classic work *General Psychopathology* (Jaspers 1997 [1959]). There he literally divides psychiatry up into these two groupings. In an era of scientific positivism, he mainly did so, again, to point out that there was a space for *Verstehen* in psychiatry, that not everything could be comprehended with a purely *Erklären* approach.

One can see the contours of Dilthey's thinking (especially the triad of lived experience, expressions, and synthetic meaning) in Jaspers's work. First there is empathy; Jaspers clearly emphasized this aspect of *Verstehen* in much more detail than Dilthey (whose "lived experience" was important but not as central for Jaspers). This may simply reflect their different subject matters; with psychiatric patients, empathy was central. For Dilthey, with historical questions (and not simply historical figures), it was less so. Second, Jaspers placed great emphasis on dialogue, on the interchange between doctor and patient. The psychiatrist would try hard to empathize, to understand the first person experience of the patient, through the open work of dialogue. Communication became, in fact, a central feature of Jaspers's mature philosophy (including his work on religion). In interviewing psychiatric patients, the concept of "expressions" translated into communication or dialogue. For Dilthey, studying the past, expressions were to be found in documents and letters. The last part of Dilthey's triad is found everywhere in Jaspers— not only in the subjective perspective of the patient as to the nature of one's experience of psychopathology but also in the psychiatrist's effort to derive some meaning from the patient's experiences, to pull together all the strands of his psychopathology into some meaningful understanding. For Jaspers, this last step became a diagnostic hallmark of psychosis, if, after all the hard work of empathy and communication, the psychiatrist failed to understand any meaning at all in the individual's experiences (the "un-Understandibility" criterion for delusions). *Verstehen* played out in Jaspers's approach to psychiatry by emphasizing empathy, dialogue, trying to appreciate the first-person subjective experiences of the person one is treating, and attending to the subjective meaning of psychopathology.

Method-Based Psychiatry Today
Leston Havens and the Harvard School

The ground-breaking work of Jaspers had impact in Germany and in the United Kingdom and some parts of Latin America (such as Chile) but little effect in the rest of the psychiatric world, especially in the United States. His work was not translated into English until 1963, and the first article on him in an American psychiatric journal was written in 1967 by Leston Havens, a prominent Harvard psychiatric teacher and psychotherapist (Havens 1967). Soon thereafter Havens was the first to apply and extend his ideas to American psychiatry as a whole, in his book *Approaches to the Mind* (Havens 1987 [1973]). Though not doing so explicitly, Havens essentially used the *Erklären* and *Verstehen* concepts as applied to schools of psychiatry: *Erklären* became the "objective-descriptive school" as exemplified by Kraepelin, using empirical methods of observation, description, and biological causation. *Verstehen* was reflected in three schools: the *psychoanalytic,* exemplified by Freud, using the methods of free association and transference interpretation augmented by a specific theory of psychology; the *existential,* exemplified by Jaspers, using the methods of empathy and "putting the world in brackets" (the method of the philosopher Edmund Husserl); and the *interpersonal/social,* exemplified by Harry Stack Sullivan, Erik Erikson, and others, using methods that converged on the real interpersonal relationship (rather than inferred intrapsychic structures) or on social relations. Confusion in psychiatry, argued Havens, stemmed from applying only one method to all aspects of the field (dogmatism) or from applying any and all methods willy-nilly (eclecticism). Havens was the first thinker in psychiatry to use the term *pluralism* defined to contrast it with eclecticism (see glossary: an application of the right school for the appropriate condition or topic; being neither dogmatic nor eclectic). This pluralism is clearly the same idea as what I term *method-based psychiatry,* the notion that Jaspers put forward when he said that psychiatry needed to use both *Erklären* and *Verstehen* methods within its scope, not to mix the two, nor to just use one approach. The method-based concept is the basis for Dilthey's critique of positivism in science and in history, Weber's critique of positivism in sociology, and William James and Charles Peirce's critique of positivism in philosophy.

Paul McHugh and the Johns Hopkins School

A decade later, the *Erklären-Verstehen* insight was taken up by the leaders of the Johns Hopkins University department of psychiatry, Paul McHugh and Phillip Slavney, and through their pedagogical and political efforts, this approach has informed the education of generations of psychiatrists in that institution.[4] In *The Perspectives of Psychiatry* (McHugh and Slavney 1998 [1983]), McHugh and Slavney were the first in American psychiatry to explicitly acknowledge their debt to Jaspers and to the *Erklären-Verstehen* concept, which they updated in a way this is different from (and in many ways complementary to) Havens: *Verstehen* was termed the "life story" perspective—a frankly hermeneutic concept about how individuals can ascribe meaning (rightly or wrongly) to their experiences; the work of psychotherapy (influenced especially by the ideas of Jerome Frank [J. D. Frank and Frank 1991]) was seen as the construction of heuristic meanings that might help patients. The truth or falsity of those meanings was less at issue than their pragmatic value: did they help people feel and live better and more happily? *Erklären* was divided into three parts: the "disease" perspective, which corresponds to the classic biomedical model of observing signs and symptoms, defining syndromes, and looking for biological etiologies to those syndromes; the "behavior" perspective, which seeks to explain motivated behaviors, the doing of things for reasons, like obtaining pleasure or avoiding pain; and the "dimensional" perspective, which explains how conditions or behaviors reflect more or less susceptibility to them (as opposed to the categorical presence or absence of a disease).

McHugh and Slavney further related each perspective to specific conditions: thus schizophrenia and manic-depressive illness were best understood by the disease model, addictions with the behavior perspective, personality conditions with the dimensional perspective, and mild to moderate anxiety or neurotic unhappiness with the life story perspective.

The Emptiness of the Biopsychosocial Model

What a rich mass of ideas exist on which modern psychiatry can draw, beyond the pale recitation of the need for "biological, psychological, and social" aspects to medicine! Perhaps George Engel, and probably Roy Grinker, would have agreed with the utility of the *Verstehen* concept in medicine and psychiatry. Engel interpreted it narrowly, though; he was anxious to include the sciences of psychology and sociology and public health into medicine, but he wanted to keep out those dangerous "arts": and art, poetry, and literature was not science and thus not relevant.

Dilthey, in contrast, greatly valued poetry as an important aspect of the knowledge of *Verstehen*. Famous for planning multivolume books, of which he published only the first, one of Dilthey's few completed works during his lifetime was a treatise called *Poetik* (Dilthey 1985). He especially was impressed by the figure of Johann Wolfgang von Goethe and the deep wisdom of his poetry. This relevance of poetry and the humanities was a key aspect of Dilthey's view of *Verstehen* (other thinkers like William James would be sympathetic to Dilthey on this topic). For Engel, though, poetry and the arts were meaningless, at least as far as medicine and psychiatry were concerned.

This is curious. Near the end of his life, Engel responded in writing to a manuscript on the relevance of ideal types to diagnosis (Schwartz and Wiggins 1987). There, Schwartz and Wiggins identified *Verstehen* with the view of idiographic knowledge, the concept of the uniqueness of individuals and events (Rickert's concept, which Dilthey resisted). They contrasted this knowledge with nomologic, or general, laws, and they asserted that empirical psychiatry had taken the nomologic approach exclusively, in keeping with the logical positivism popular in philosophy of science in the 1950s and earlier (especially in the work of the philosopher Carl Hempel [1965]). They argued that biological psychiatry was faulty because it took this positivistic approach and contrasted it with a nonpositivistic view of science, such as Max Weber's work on ideal types. After sending their manuscript to Engel, they received comments from him, which they included in the published article as follows: "Idiographic investigations characterize what every physician does with each patient, and thus defines what characterizes the nature of the scientific work of the clinician, irrespective of his discipline" (p. 289). Schwartz and Wiggins then relate their rejection of positivism in psychiatry to an embracing of Engel's biopsychosocial model. I do not see how the former entails the latter, however, because many other options exist beside this model. Engel explicitly rejected the humanities and poetry. It is hard to comprehend this rejection, given that poetry is sometimes defined and defended as a reflection of the unique and the unrepeatable in human experience (Eastman 1921; Ros-Zanet 2004)—idiographic reality. One would think, if Engel took the idiographic nature of each person's reality seriously, that he would embrace, like William Osler, how literature and poetry provide background wisdom with which clinicians would be better equipped to relate to each patient. A psychiatrist recently explained the clinical need for the humanities this way (Geppert 2008): If you are treating an older person from the deep South, prior reading of Walker Percy or William Faulkner might allow you to better connect to that person's sensibilities and sensitivities. Engel would rather replace such wisdom with "knowledge," based on the brilliant insights of a Victorian Viennese clinician, about how unconscious defense mechanisms might drive behavior. As helpful as those insights might be, there is something to be said for Goethe's wisdom too, as Freud, winner of the Goethe prize and a great admirer of the poet, would be the first to acknowledge.

Despite his protestations to the contrary, Engel still lived with a pinched definition of science, not as painfully narrow as pure positivism, but hardly profound. He failed to appreciate how much one can use *Verstehen* as a valid method of knowledge, as a science, in human studies, even in literature. And he failed to appreciate the limits of *Verstehen*—why some kinds of purported scientific knowledge, like his beloved psychosomatic psychoanalysis, were hardly scientific.

Engel called science things that were not science, and he called nonscience things that are science. He was not the last word, and not even the first word, in the work of bringing *Verstehen* to medicine and psychiatry; and his biopsychosocial model is a weak and poor vessel for breaking free from positivism. It is time to turn elsewhere, and we have a rich and deep scientific and philosophical tradition to which we can turn.

Perhaps now we can find a new path away from dogmatisms, while avoiding the mire of biopsychosocial eclecticism. Maybe there is another way.

A Pluralist Case Conference

In 2004, I helped organize a "pluralistic case conference" at Cambridge Hospital, in Massachusetts, which was conducted by Leston Havens and Alfred Marguelis, both prominent psychoanalytically trained psychotherapists who also have existential leanings (Havens 2005; Marguelis 1989). A psychology intern presented the case of a 17-year-old working-class young man who conflicted with his mother and siblings. (His father had long left the family.) He recently also had been drawn into a violent fight between his friends and a rival group and came to treatment for depressive symptoms and suicidal thoughts. Over the past year, the intern had sought to engage him in psychotherapy using "interpretive" methods, derived from psychoanalytic concepts: he sought to indicate to the young man that his thoughts of self-harm might reflect internally directed wishes to harm others, such as those who had attacked him and his friends, or perhaps feelings of anger toward his absent father. Yet, he seemed "resistant" to these interpretations, and no meaningful progress seemed to be happening, despite the earnest best efforts of the intern and the close supervision of a number of experienced psychoanalytically oriented psychotherapists. The teen also had begun treatment with a psychiatric resident, who had diagnosed major depressive disorder and prescribed fluoxetine (Prozac). Despite adequate dosages, which were increased after nonresponse, for more than six months, he showed minimal improvement in depressive symptoms.

In the discussion that followed, both Havens and Marguelis emphasized the need to first connect with the young man, through an existential common ground, rather than seeking to engage in psychoanalytic interpretations. I added that the diagnosis of "major depression," and treatment with antidepressant, seemed superficial. What was his main problem? What method would best identify the source of his problems? What method would be the best single initial treatment for him? Neither the psychology intern, nor his supervisors, nor the psychiatric resident and his supervisors, had asked any of these questions. They seemed to simply take it for granted that it would be fine to take a psychoanalytic orientation with the patient, in the case of the psychotherapy approach taken, or that it would be fine to take a biomedical orientation with him, in the case of the psychopharmacology approach taken. It was also assumed that the combination of both approaches was acceptable, without asking why.

The biopsychosocial model, by allowing all permutations of causes and treatments, allows one to avoid such questions. In contrast, a noneclectic method-based psychiatry would force one to ask those questions, to choose one method, with justification for why it is to be preferred to others, and then to pursue it purely. In this case, the discussants thought that the young man initially needed to be approached from the existential method. They felt that we did not clearly understand what was going on in his life, why he felt the way he did, how he felt about his peers, his father, his mother, his enemies—his world. They believed that until we understood the experience of the person being treated, we could not draw any conclusions about whether any psychoanalytic interpretations would be warranted, or whether he indeed had the kind of symptoms and course consistent with a biologically based disease entity like unipolar depression, or whether medication treatment would be necessary, and, if so, which exact medications would be best to use. An existentially oriented psychotherapy, without any medications, and without any psychoanalytic interpretations, for six months or longer, was the recommendation, a method-based conclusion that weighed all the possibilities and picked one perspective as the most plausible.

It could be that existential psychotherapy, the one pure method best suited to that individual's situation, would be both curative as well as diagnostic; it might be all that was required. Or it could be that existential psychotherapy would reveal that he, diagnostically, indeed had a severe mood disorder, at which point appropriate medications could be instituted. That would be an example of sequential use of multiple methods.

One might or might not agree with the method-based interpretation suggested, but its advantages over the failure of the biopsychosocial model in this case may be apparent.

Antieclectic Method-Based Psychiatry

The reader may recall that Grinker held the view that "one can learn more about interrelations between somatic and psychic or between psychic and social systems by making observations *at the boundaries of their intersections*" (Grinker 1975; italics in original). Thus, Grinker emphasized the relevance of knowledge at the boundaries of disciplines and methods, rather than from within methods, a multidisciplinary eclecticism that went beyond George Engel's additive eclecticism, the view that the different methods or disciplines or perspectives could be added together to provide the best overall knowledge (the more, the better). The kind of method-based psychiatry suggested here differs from eclecticism: unlike the view of Roy Grinker, method-based psychiatry views the most valid knowledge as occurring within a single method; unlike the theory of George Engel, method-based psychiatry thinks that the addition of methods confuses, rather than clarifies: it is like diluting water with other agents—pure water is preferable. This method-based view accepts something that Grinker and Engel both rejected, something that dogmatists like Freud and Kraepelin understood: a single method, purely and appropriately applied, produces the most accurate knowledge. Yet such a method-based approach differs from dogmatism by denying that any single method is sufficient for all of psychiatry. Grinker, much more than Engel, verged at times on a more profound and less eclectic view; when discussing the need to pay attention to more than one method or discipline in psychiatry, he wrote that a psychiatrist "need not have a highly specialized knowledge of more than one discipline. He needs to know, however, the extent of his own field, its boundaries beyond which he cannot skillfully reach where he requires other professional help in multidisciplinary operations" (Grinker 1975). (See the glossary for more distinctions between a method-based pluralistic approach versus eclecticism.)

Though such a method-based framework for psychiatry has long existed, it was overshadowed by the simplistic and comfortable certainties of the dogmas of psychiatry, and it was completely ignored by the eclectic theories of Adolf Meyer, Grinker, and Engel. The hard work of reanalyzing and reinterpreting those approaches, while avoiding the trap of eclecticism, is a task that remains for our field. A good source from which to begin this important work, extended in the next chapter to defining mental illness, can be found in the efforts of Karl Jaspers, supplanted by a rediscovery of the medical humanism tradition of William Osler.

CHAPTER SEVENTEEN

A New Psychiatric Humanism

We may end this book with three key questions that the biopsychosocial model sought and, in my view, failed to answer: What is illness? What is health? What is the proper role of medicine as a profession?

A common view is that medicine is a purely biological discipline, with no need to attend to mental matters or the individual as a person or anything apart from the diseased body. This is the so-called biomedical model, the dehumanized cold approach that is often criticized. The focus is on disease; all else is ignored. Psychiatry, on this view, is an almost spiritual profession, not part of medicine, but there to handle behavioral problems that cannot be explained physically. This would seem to be an extreme, and hardly defensible, position. Yet as a practicing doctor, I can claim, unscientifically, based on anecdotal experience, that a good chunk of practicing doctors think this way today, and a probably larger chunk have always thought this way. This view is in fact consistent with the basic philosophy of medicine underlying Thomas Szasz's view of mental illness as a myth (Szasz 1984 [1960]). This view of medicine is also the straw man called "biomedical reductionism," which exists in reality, it is true, but which also exists for academic sport—as something to attack on the part of postmodernists of all stripes, along with advocates of the biopsychosocial approach. There is much noise and debate, but little clarity.

Here again I will turn to the work of Karl Jaspers to analyze different models of health, illness, and medicine, and to see if he can point us to a solution.[1]

A Biological Existentialist

Jaspers is widely seen as a holistic thinker. His emphasis on the human subject and on the limits of empirical science is often seen as implying an eclectic perspective. This interpretation of his thinking has especially taken root in those who approach his work on psychiatry from familiarity with his existentialist philosophical writings. The existentialist perspective privileges the individual, and when applied to medicine and psychiatry, it would seem logical that it should privilege the individual person or case over any emphasis on diseases or theories.

This ethereal spiritualist antibiological Jaspers is, in my view, a misreading of his thinking. I believe that a basic key to understanding Jaspers is the concept of methodological consciousness, the notion that one must pay attention to one's methods in science, in medicine, and in psychiatry, that between fact and method no sharp line can be drawn, that no single method can be applied to all cases, but that there are better or worse methods (based on each method's strengths and limitations) that justify using one and not another for a specific condition or case (Ghaemi 2003). This is the method-based epistemology that underlies Jaspers's classic work, *General Psychopathology* (Jaspers 1997 [1959]), where he applies the two methods of *Erklären* and *Verstehen* to psychiatry. This basic concept underlies all his thinking, making him a *biological existentialist*.

Defining Health and Illness

In discussing the meaning of health and illness, Jaspers first notes that value judgments are unavoidable. This perspective automatically negates the positivistic or Szaszian view that physical illness is a fact, while mental "illnesses" are cultural values. Just as, in contemporary philosophy, the distinction between fact and value has been increasingly questioned, so in understanding the concept of illness, value must be allowed a role. Contemporary philosophizing agrees with where Jaspers was in 1913, when he wrote *General Psychopathology*.

The fact that values inhere in medical illness does not imply that all such illness is a myth of social construction. Rather, values are inherent in all human phenomena, including health and illness. Values are present in how we perceive pain or why we decide to go to doctors or not. Values are part of the illness process, but it does not follow that illnesses are *nothing but* values (Fulford 1989). So the first step invalidates positivism but does not entail postmodernism (or its twin: eclecticism). Jaspers goes on to describe health as "a normative biological concept," which is not, however, clearly articulated. This brings us to the question of how health and illness should be understood relative to each other. There seem to be two basic perspectives: either health is absence of illness (the narrow view, as described in psychiatry by Aubrey Lewis) or illness is absence of health (the broad view, as advocated in psychiatry by Leston Havens; Ghaemi 2003).

The Pathologization of Health

Most physicians are inclined to view illness on its own terms, as a morbid process, without feeling a need to previously define health. There are many problems with this view, much discussed in the postmodernist literature. In psychiatry, Leston Havens has made informed critiques of this perspective, pointing out that this approach leads to overpathologization (Havens 1984). You can read entire psychiatric hospital charts, he notes, and never find a single piece of good news! All aspects of patients' lives are viewed as illness. As noted previously, even the words we use are totalistic: the patient *is* schizophrenic; he *is* depressed; she *is* bipolar. If we view illness as something that happens *to* otherwise healthy patients, we would use the verb "to have": The patient *has* bipolar disorder, but otherwise does not have a whole host of other entities, and, by the way, the bipolar disorder only affects part of his psyche, not all of it. Havens makes the point that general medicine is much less pathologizing than psychiatry: when we go to the internist, we get some tests, the vast majority of which are normal, and we are reassured by those results. If a single result out of many is abnormal, we understanding the possibility of isolated illness in the larger context of greater health. In contrast, he argues, when was the last time a patient went to a psychiatrist and was told he was perfectly fine? Havens suggests that psychiatry will not advance diagnostically until tests of normal functioning are developed, analogous to the reflex hammer and the tuning fork in neurological diagnosis.

Havens's critique is convincing, but defining illness on the basis of health produces more problems than it solves. This approach shifts the burden to defining what health is, and there are as many different views about the nature of health as there are about the nature of illness.

The World Health Organization Definition

One might begin with the "official" definition of health, that of the World Health Organization: "a state of complete, physical, mental, and social well-being and not merely the absence of disease or infirmity." Psychiatrist Aubrey Lewis has demolished this view as empty verbiage (Lewis 1967):[2]

> A proposition could hardly be more comprehensive than that, or more meaningless. But to condemn it because it is meaningless is to ignore the history and complexity of the idea behind it . . . an ancient formula of unattainable wholeness of body, mind and soul, realized in the Golden Age but long since forfeited. . . . Now if the various organs work well enough not to draw attention to themselves, and their owner is free from pain or discomfort, he usually supposes that he is in good health. The criterion is then a subjective one. But if he avails himself of the mass X-ray service and in consequence learns that his lung shows strong evidence of tuberculous diseases, he ceases to consider that he is in good health: the criterion he now adopts is an extraneous one, *viz.*, the assertion of a physician who relies on objective or pathological data. It is evident that the physician's criteria of physical health are not the same as the patient's, and that, in practice, it is the presence of disease that can be recognized, not the presence of health. There are no positive indications of health which can be relied on, and we consider everyone healthy who is free from any evidence of disease or infirmity.

Three Concepts of Health

Lewis's critique is consistent with Jaspers's thinking. Jaspers identified three basic concepts of health, all of which he considered inadequate: (1) the ancient Greek notion of health as "harmony of opposing forces," or being "midway between opposites" (associated with Galen in Roman and later eras); (2) the Hellenistic notion of health as the highest value, with the Epicureans wishing "contentment with a measured satisfaction of [reduced] needs" and the Stoics wanting to "destroy all passions for *ataraxia* [equanimity];" and (3) modern views of health as "self-realization." Twentieth-century philosophers, such as Martha Nussbaum (1996), have resuscitated interest in the last two notions, with self-realization being connected to Aristotle's notion of *eudemonia* ("flourishing"). Like Nussbaum, Jaspers describes how the Hellenistic philosophies were "a kind of therapy." The corresponding views of illness that derive from these concepts of health are (1) disharmony or "disintegration into opposites;" (2) having too much affect or passion; and (3) "dis-ingenuousness" or "flight into illness" (as proposed by psychoanalysis). Jaspers cites Nietzsche to claim that the first two notions bring about "an impoverishment of the psyche," and he judges the third viewpoint to be empty (what it means to be "self-realized" is vague).

To get beyond this dilemma, Jaspers emphasizes that we need to fully appreci-ate the value-based nature of assessments of health and illness. He comments that we either base health on value norms or statistical norms. The value norm, based on some kind of "ideal concept," seems more common than mere statistical norms, partly because the statistical average may not always seem "good." He might have cited the psychoanalytic dictum that we are all neurotic, some more so than oth-ers (or as the old saying, often attributed to an unknown Quaker, goes: "Everyone is mad except for me and thee, and I am not so sure about thee."). Or he might have appreciated the medical observation that certain features, like height, weight, and blood pressure, vary greatly from culture to culture, thus challenging definitions of what is normal or abnormal. If "the average, that is, the attribute of the majority, is the measure for health," "therefore slight feeblemindedness . . . [or neurosis, or slightly high blood pressure or slightly low height] is what is healthy. But slight feeblemindedness is a term for something 'sick.' Therefore something that is sick is also normal. Therefore healthy = sick" (1997 [1959], p. 784). The statistical aver-age does not provide a means of defining illness and health without the use of value judgments.

Insight

Next we arrive at the problem of inserting a human being into this picture, a per-son with feelings about whatever may be happening in his body. "The individual feels himself to be ill, knows or wants to know his illness, and adopts an attitude to his illness" (p. 782). The introduction of awareness ("insight" in the terminology of psychopathology) leads to two types of false presentations that cloud our under-standing of illness. There is the *false negative,* somebody is ill but does not realize that he is so: "There is . . . somatic finding without any awareness of illness. . . . It is only with the help of the doctor's judgment that he can reach any medical in-sight." And there is the *false positive;* somebody thinks he is ill but is not: "there are feelings of illness without any objective finding. . . . The doctor finds nothing, calls them 'nervy' and dispatches them to the psychiatrist" (pp. 782–83). This happens in medicine, but it happens more in psychiatry: "With the psychic disorders the matter is altogether different and we are presented with a real problem. Either there is no somatic finding at all or the inappropriateness of the patient's attitude is part of the illness or there may be specific symptoms arising from a determination to be ill." Lack of insight is part of mania and schizophrenia, and feigned symptoms can occur with malingering or drug-seeking. Even when real mental illness occurs, somatic findings do not exist to help the practitioner. Defining illness is tough in medicine and extremely hard in psychiatry.

The Benefits of Mental Illness

Mental illness poses a further problem in that it is not merely a deficiency, something purely negative, but it can have positive aspects, as with the creativity of famous mentally ill persons. "Analytic pathographies of outstanding personalities have shown that illness not only interrupts and destroys, but that something is achieved in spite of it and even more that it can be the actual condition for certain performances." What is special to humankind—the higher faculties—predisposes us to mental illness: "It is not mere chance therefore that poets have used symbols and figures of madness for the essence of human life in its highest and most horrible possibilities, in its greatness and decline." In reference to the works of both Cervantes and Shakespeare, Jaspers says that madness evokes "awe as well as horror." He quotes Plato ("A madness sent from the gods is more desirable by far than mere human reasonableness") and Nietzsche ("How pallid and ghost-like [is] . . . so-called health"; p. 786). Mental illness reveals possibilities, Jaspers concludes, both negative and positive, which the healthy person conceals from himself. The mentally ill are to be admired, not stigmatized. He approvingly quotes an asylum psychiatrist from the 1840s: "I have higher esteem for the mentally ill than for healthy persons."

The Failure of Abstract Definitions of Health and Illness

Jaspers concludes that the general concept of illness cannot be well defined, and further that we do not need it, given a pluralistic mindset: "As scientists we want to know: what kind of phenomena are possible in the human psyche? As practitioners we want to know what are the means whereby we can advance the diverse desirabilities of psychic life? For these purposes we do not need the concept of 'illness in general' at all and we now know that no such general and uniform concept exists" (pp. 784–85).

He then contrasts the unscientific notion of *being ill* with the scientific notion of *having an illness*: "The question 'is there a morbid element or not?' contains a vestige of those old ideas according to which illnesses were Beings who took possession of people. We may say: this is an event which is unfavorable from such and such point of view . . . but if we term something as morbid in a general way we are none the wiser." (In this comment, he agrees with Havens and conflicts with Engel.)

Abstract concepts of health fail, not only for understanding illness, but also for explaining the goals of treatment: "What does the doctor see as his treatment goal? 'Health' in some undefined senses. But for one person 'health' means an unthinking, optimistic steady equilibrium through life, for another it means an awareness of God's constant presence and a feeling of peace and confidence. . . . while a third person believes himself healthy when all the unhappiness of his life, the activities which he dislikes, all that is inhospitable, is covered up by deceptive ideals and fictitious explanations" (p. 802).

In the end, Jaspers believes that we cannot define health: "A precise definition of health seems pointless if the essence of man is his *incompleteness*" (italics added). With this notion of incompleteness, we are back to the inherently method-based nature of Jaspers's epistemology, where absolute knowledge is impossible.

Jaspers concludes that perhaps we cannot clearly define illness or health, alone or in relation to each other, partly because they go together—they cannot be separated; they are, in a way, the same. If illness means "living creatures living off each other" or "radical changes of environment" or "mutations," then these things happen all the time. Thus, "being ill belongs to living as such." (One might see Jaspers's own life-long and life-threatening severe lung disease as influencing his views here.) He approvingly cites Nietzsche yet again: "Healthiness as such does not exist." Jaspers continues: "Being ill is not only the lot of isolated exceptions in life but a part of living itself as an instant in its ascent and a risk to be overcome. Life proceeds by experiment and its course is at one and the same time success and failure" (p. 785).

Just as illness in general has no meaning, so too, Jaspers says (citing Griesinger) mental illness "is not a general species"; it has to be structured, ordered, into concepts. Many are not 'sick' at all, have no "morbid process," but have "some unfavourable constitutional variant"—their personality (extremes from the statistical norm)—that leads them to hospitals.

Understandability and Empathy

How, then, are we to define specific mental illnesses now that we have given up the notion of defining them based on mental health?

We start, says Jaspers, with the phenomenon of *insight*: "The concept of illness in psychiatry is characterized by the fact that the patient's attitude to his illness, his feeling of being ill, his awareness of illness, or the complete absence of both, is not something additional to be easily corrected as in the purely somatic disorders but always an integral part of the illness itself."

He then states his famous "un-understandability" criterion, which has been misunderstood by many to be seen by Jaspers as pathognomonic of mental illness (or psychosis), whereas he makes clear that it is only the *first step* to deeper understanding of the individual and the illness:

> In the observer's case the starting-point is something which cannot be meaningfully understood whether this is a disordering of the meaningful connections by abnormal mechanisms or something 'quite mad,' that is a radical breakdown of the possibilities of communication. . . . Differential diagnosis rests on distinguishing the different kinds of ununderstandability, slight symptoms which to the lay person do not appear at all morbid can be the indicators of a most serious and destructive process whereas florid phenomena (states of excitement, called furor) can be symptoms of a relatively harmless hysteria. In the patient's case, the starting point is what he suffers. . . . These starting-points for defining illness are not reliable. There is no concordance between the phenomena as first observed and the nature, severity, and trend of the disease-process. The psychopathologist, therefore, penetrates to deeper levels by a number of methodical observations and by discovering what phenomena cluster together and the way in which they run their course, etc. As a result we now find three concepts of disease. (pp. 788–89)

Here we see how Jaspers incorporated the teaching of his predecessor at Heidelberg, Emil Kraepelin: the clustering together of phenomena, their "course, etc.," these were how Kraepelin taught nosology. Jaspers did not reject this, contrary to many of his later followers in the Heidelberg school (like Kurt Schneider). Rather, Jaspers added the *Verstehen* method as a necessary predecessor to the external observations of symptoms and course that were the method of the Kraepelinian School. The two approaches, *Verstehen* and *Erklären,* go hand in hand, the one ceding way to the other as appropriate.

Using this method, Jaspers describes three kinds of mental illnesses (in a manner similar to contemporary *Diagnostic and Statistical Manual* nosologies): "(1) as a somatic process; (2) as a serious event which breaks into healthy life for the first time and procures a psychic change; a somatic base is suspected for this but as yet not known; (3) as a variation of human life far removed from the average and somehow undesired by the affected person or by his environment and therefore in need of treatment" (p. 789).

Near the end of *General Psychopathology*, Jaspers notes that mental illnesses as somatic processes reflect "the basic attitudes of medicine and the natural sciences which only accept the somatic as the decisive factor. . . . In fact there is a field of organic cerebral disease where the demand for a somatic basis can be gratified and where the psychic events are symptoms of a known physical event. But the difficulties which remain are by no means negligible. In scarcely a quarter of hospital patients do we know the organic basis for the disorder." One might comment that in Jaspers's era, most of these patients had what was then called general paralysis of the insane, known by then to be caused by neurosyphilis. This disease was treatable by 1927 with malaria therapy (the only Nobel Prize for treatment given to a psychiatrist, Julius von Wagner-Jaurregg), and cured by the 1950s with penicillin (thus the most powerful psychotropic drug ever discovered). It is noteworthy that here Jaspers flies directly in the face of postmodernism and social constructionism: some mental disorders are physical diseases; they are not all simply cultural phenomena. Jaspers obviously equally argues against a positivistic mind-brain identity.

The second category of suspected somatic illnesses are defined by their psychic (rather than unknown somatic) features, and here Jaspers places the "psychoses in the three hereditary groupings," or the main illnesses of psychiatric practice—schizophrenia and manic-depressive illness along with severe melancholia. He wishes we had identified psychic "basic functions" that are disturbed to better classify these conditions, but because those psychological functions have not been well described, he says, we have "a multitude of theories and a host of descriptions" (p. 790).

The third group consists of "the unwanted variations of human nature," in which "the concepts of natural science are indispensable but do not suffice and everywhere we find a gulf between man and beast." These represent the personality conditions, extremes on normal personality traits.

One way to summarize mental illnesses might be to conflate these three categories to two: biological illnesses (the known or suspected somatic forms) and problems of living (either due to personality extremes or simply due to extreme life events or a combination of the two). Using Jaspers's method-based approach, the first type of illness may be best analyzed with *Erklären* and is best treated with somatic means (medications); the second type of illness is best understood with *Verstehen* and is best treated either outside of the medical field (through religious, spiritual, or other psychic means) or through psychotherapies. In either case, treatment of some kind is given, but the right kind of treatment needs to be chosen for the right kind of condition (which I label method-based psychiatry).

Existential Psychotherapy

Jaspers's discussion of health and illness moves on to the final section of *General Psychopathology,* called "The Meaning of Medical Practice" (pp. 790–822). Most of this section is actually given to explaining the nature of psychotherapy, perhaps because the more traditional concepts of somatic medical practice were viewed by him as already well known, while psychotherapy was a novel concept in his era.

In medical practice, he contrasts the two extremes of "therapeutic nihilism" and "therapeutic overenthusiasm," the first overrelying on knowledge for its own sake and seeing medicine as a pure science instead of as an art, the second believing wrongly that "something should be done or attempted in all circumstances" and that "practice only needs aptitude, not knowledge." Jaspers would come out on the side of the hard-headed proponents of evidence-based medicine in today's debates about the role of science in medicine: "In the long run . . . effective practice can only be based on the certainties of knowledge." Practice needs to depend on science, on real knowledge, not just experience. Yet practice, while dependent on science for its methods, has to look elsewhere for its aims. Its goals, its view of health and illness, are based on its values; science cannot provide those values. Practitioners of psychiatry needed to pay attention to their own value systems in the course of giving treatments. Why are they giving treatments? What goals are they pursuing? They should not cover up these values with scientific pseudoexplanations.

"Things are expected from science which it cannot provide. In this age of superstitious belief in science, science is used to conceal unanswerable facts. . . . A form of pseudoscience may be used to express something that is by no means known but only wished for." Jaspers is especially making this point in relation to psychotherapies, which enact value systems to a much greater extent than does somatic medicine.

He then goes into an analysis of what is entailed in psychotherapies, concluding that the root of all of them is the relationship between the therapist and the person seeking treatment, which again connects psychotherapies to all medical therapy, because that relationship is always present, even in somatic treatments. In psychotherapies, the entirety of the treatment is that relationship: "What is left as the ultimate thing in the doctor-patient relationship is existential communication, which goes far beyond anything that can be planned or methodically staged. The whole treatment is thus absorbed and defined within a community of two selves who live at the possibilities of Existence itself, as reasonable beings. . . . Doctor and patient are both human beings and as such are fellow-travellers in destiny. . . . There is no final solution."

Here is how Jaspers concludes his magnum opus: Psychiatric treatment ranges on a spectrum where "the widest polarities lie in whether a doctor turns to what can be discovered by science, that is to the biological event, or whether he turns to the freedom of man." The distinction is essential, and it is not a matter of preference. Where biological disease is present, existential empathy with human freedom has no place and vice versa. The doctor needs to know which method to use and when, and he needs to know how to use both methods. One approach involves treating with drugs, the other requires existential collaboration. "Life I can treat," Jaspers concludes, "but to freedom I can only appeal."

How Would Jaspers Practice Psychiatry Today?

By discussing existential methods in psychotherapy, Jaspers is addressing the key problem with defining illnesses without defining health: the risk of overpathologizing, overdiagnosis, social construction, and abuse of medical power. The corrective to these risks is to remember that diseases, though real objective entities in the natural world, happen to individual human beings, free men and women, with *feelings* about having or not having a disease. And, sometimes, there is no disease at all, but only problems of individual free human beings, in which case—using method-based psychiatry—the disease model does not apply.

Thus, today, if Jaspers were active as a psychiatrist, he would be prescribing medications for diseases such as schizophrenia and bipolar disorder, and even severe depression, but he would also be cognizant of the positive aspects of mental illness and of the many presentations of psychopathology that do not have biological roots. He would also disparage the dogmatic oversimplification of those who think that, because *some* psychopathology is nonbiological, then *all* (or most) psychopathology must be nonbiological.

The Medical Humanism of Osler and Jaspers

In the end, Jaspers promoted a method-based psychiatry that was nothing more or less than a proper understanding of science applied to psychiatry and medicine. His views were completely in keeping with the work of William Osler and with the concept of medical humanism. One takes a biologically reductionist model of disease and applies it where appropriate, but always with a humanistic awareness of the importance of the person, the individual, who has the disease. No disease wipes out the person, and no understanding of person is adequate by itself when a bodily disease is present. I will reiterate that this is not new—merely forgotten. Osler resuscitated the Hippocratic view that medicine consisted of three factors: the patient, the disease, and the doctor; an idea that had been lost under two millennia of subservience to Galen's theory of health and illness. For centuries humoral dogma—the belief that illness was an imbalance of humors, or fluids—had been enough—no talk of persons and diseases and doctors was needed. After the Galenic theory was proven wrong, Osler took modern medicine back to the ethically and scientifically sound Hippocratic approach.

This humanism is individual and existential; it is not captured by another scientific discipline (like psychology or sociology) tacked onto the discipline of biology (as George Engel argued), and thus the biopsychosocial model does not do it justice. It is not captured by any single nonbiological theory of medicine or psychiatry (e.g., psychoanalysis). It is best understood through an understanding of literature, to the uniqueness of humanity and of each individual human being, which is best approached, though never completely captured, in poetry and fiction.

Recall that Osler divided medical knowledge into two parts: scientific and humanistic. The scientific part related to diseases and was based on the sciences of pathology, laboratory medicine, and clinical observation. The humanistic part related to understanding the persons who had diseases and was based on literary wisdom and worldly experience with the feelings and wishes of human beings.

None of this entails a dismissal of science—of positivism, yes, but not of science proper. For medicine, in Osler's view, was an art based on a science; not just an art, and not just a science. Without science, medicine would be empty; without art, it would be irrelevant. Despite the claims of postmodernism, Osler offered another choice: he rejected a cold inhumane approach to medicine, but he offered the biomedical model plus the art of medicine as an alternative.

Karl Jaspers's method-based psychiatry also leads to this conclusion; he did for psychiatry what Osler did for medicine, though Jaspers emphasized an existential-ist philosophy as something in addition to literature that would provide the humanistic element needed for psychiatric practice.

His existentialism was a *biological existentialism,* not a social constructionist, postmodernist, antimedical perspective. (Jaspers was not Heidegger.) Too often, phenomenology and existentialism get conflated with antiscience and nonbiological perspectives in medicine and psychiatry. This need not be the case, and this approach is certainly different from what Jaspers stood for. In medicine and psychiatry we need to be biological, because we are dealing with physical diseases, but we also need to be existential, because we are dealing with individual persons (whether they have diseases or problems of living). The two perspectives are not opposite or exclusive, as many seem to assume.

The Jaspersian/Oslerian option would allow us to keep the standard scientific model of biomedicine while emphasizing a humanistic and existential orientation to the needs, values, and desires of individual human beings. This is not to say that scientific research in psychology and social sciences may not aid such person-based approaches but rather that such scientific work will not exhaust the complexity of humanity. At some level, we would have to admit that human beings cannot be completely captured by the methods of science, that there is another kind of knowledge—literary, philosophical, intuitive—that can inform us about our lives and our loves. Without needing to add the biopsychosocial model or psychoanalytic theory or other philosophical or psychological dogmas, we can add a humanistic wisdom rooted in Socrates and Hippocrates, Shakespeare and Cervantes, Goethe and Nietzsche, William James and Walker Percy, James Joyce and Rainer Maria Rilke, and William Faulkner and even Jalaluldin Rumi. What an excellent medical model—and what an excellent vision of psychiatry—that would be.

Afterword

Pre-empting the Straw Man

There is one reaction to this book that I expect to receive, based on my discussions about it with many colleagues. My criticisms of the biopsychosocial (BPS) model may be granted, but it will be argued that these relate only to the "old" model of George Engel; the "new and improved" versions that exist now would survive my critiques. This is a version of the "straw man" argument: weak or simplified versions of an idea are set up and then attacked, thereby seeking to reject stronger versions of the idea indirectly and by association.

Engel's BPS model is not a straw man version; it is the classic version. Being classic, it deserves respect, and so does this critique of it. I have not put words in the mouths of Engel and Roy Grinker; extensive direct quotations are provided, and I have used all of their primary published works, as well as most available secondary sources.

It is not exactly the same to claim the straw man argument and to say that newer versions of the model are better. The straw man argument involves actual oversimplification: this book documents the classic work of Grinker and Engel such that this criticism cannot apply. The new-and-improved argument implies that what is newer is better and unrelated to what preceded it. Such apologists for the BPS model would have to claim that current views can be upheld completely separate from, and unrelated to, the views of Engel and Grinker. This kind of thinking is clearly apologetics, an attempt to defend an opinion at all costs, and is simply illogical. It would be like claiming that one could be a Marxist and have nothing to do with Marx or a psychoanalyst with no relation to Freud. Obviously, many newer versions of Marxism are different from Marx's own viewpoint and, similarly, newer ("eclectic") versions of psychoanalysis may diverge from Freud. Yet the progenitors cannot be completely disowned; the sins of the fathers are visited on the sons.

This is not to say that no improvements can be made, or have been made, on the BPS model. Let me be clear: this book criticizes BPS eclecticism but it does not thereby seek to uphold biological dogmatism. I explicitly reject all kinds of dogmatism, whether biological or psychoanalytic, at the same time as rejecting eclecticism. I am seeking an antieclectic, antidogmatic way of thinking for psychiatry. This is what I mean by method-based psychiatry. Someone else may try to improve BPS eclecticism by making it less eclectic: Let us suppose BPS revisionists were to conclude that *not* all mental illness *always* has biological, psychological, and social factors; that it is legitimate at times to take a purely biological or a purely social approach to a condition; that simply mixing and adding methods does not inherently improve our knowledge; and that *sometimes* pure reductionism is appropriate for certain illnesses or conditions. If all these perspectives were accepted, and revisionists wanted to call it a new-and-improved BPS model, they could do so, but why use the term *biopsychosocial* at all? Why not call it something else, for reasons both conceptual and historical: conceptually, this amount of revision converts the BPS concept into something quite different from what its originators intended (it would be like insisting that the graduated income tax is a type of Marxism);[1] historically, this kind of perspective was long upheld, when Engel and Grinker were schoolchildren, by Karl Jaspers. Would not historical accuracy instead support using terms that Jaspers promoted before the notion of biopsychosocial was conceived of, terms related to his "methodological consciousness"?

I have come to a conclusion. Many mental health professionals, and others interested in psychiatry (in the social sciences and humanities), are averse to rejecting the BPS concept because they want to reject biological dogmatism. Everybody hates the idea that mental illness can be reduced to the brain and drugs; nobody wants this, perhaps because of some wish to preserve space for the soul, and a larger sense of humanity, in our self-image. Even though I am not sure why this concern should exist (are we lesser humans because much of psychosis turned out to be neurosyphilis?), I can sympathize with it. I want to reject biological dogmatism, too. BPS sympathizers need to hear that rejection of their model does not entail that everyone needs to run to the local pharmacy to obtain lifetime prescriptions for Prozac. There are other options besides dehumanized biological reductionism and the BPS model.

The proponents of the new-and-improved apology also need to explain just where these kinder, gentler versions of the BPS model are to be found. They have to explain what there is beyond the current BPS perspectives provided by Engel's actual disciples in Rochester, by an international group with a public health orientation in the United Kingdom, and by recent philosophically oriented defenses (all reviewed and critiqued in chapter 5 and later chapters). Those newer versions are much like the classic ones in many ways and, as described in this book, are hardly improved. Those who would simply assert that there are better BPS versions need to respond to the specific critiques I have made of those candidates.

If I had to pick one of the BPS-like candidates that would seem to be among the stronger options, I would look at the profession of public health, especially work on the association between social factors and health. Poverty and social class, for instance, are likely related to risk for many chronic medical conditions, such as diabetes and cardiovascular disease. The field of social epidemiology, which has arisen in the past decade or so, has begun to study the concept of "social capital," defined as how cohesiveness in a community seems to be associated with better health (Berkman and Kawachi 2000). Grounded in the early work of sociologist Emile Durkheim on suicide, this field is promising, but it is new, and research in it has only just begun. Evidence also exists against the social capital / health connection (Kushner and Sterk 2005), and we should be wary of wholeheartedly accepted socially oriented public health as the long awaited, new-and-improved BPS approach. Some public health scholars have made the connection between their field and the BPS model. Yet the BPS approach is itself thinly coherent, as described in this book, and many aspects of social epidemiology are only beginning to be understood. Certainly, as an overarching theory for medicine or psychiatry, public health and social epidemiology do not provide a new and improved substitute for the biopsychosocial model.

To summarize, the BPS model has never been a scientific model or even a philosophically coherent model. It was a slogan whose ultimate basis was eclecticism. And eclecticism was meant to free practitioners to do what they pleased, which in our day means freedom to reject biological reductionism. Today, this eclectic goal dovetails dangerously with a strong and powerful force in our culture and in the social sciences: postmodernism. Postmodernists believe in social construction: to them everything, including all science, is socially relative. The BPS eclectics and the postmodernists both wish to emphasize the psychological or the social at the expense of the biological. The danger is that they no longer see social factors as factors but as all there is. They fail to take biology seriously (Kushner 2006) and begin to deconstruct even the most biological of mental illnesses, like manic-depressive illness, into nothingness (Healy 2007).[2] They may also pay lip service to the biology of mental illnesses but then talk about nothing but social construction. Can we not avoid both cultural reductionism and biological reductionism? It is a strength, not a weakness, of science (and medicine and psychiatry) that it is aware of its tentativeness, that it is self-critical, and that it recognizes that truth is corrected error (Kushner 1998). The existence of truths, indeed truths of biology, beyond all social construction is what is at issue. Most BPS eclectics deny this view or act as if it were untrue; so do postmodernists. We need not be biological reductionists to accept the biological reality of some mental illnesses and the relevance of social and psychological factors for them; and we need not be cultural reductionists to recognize the pure social construction of other mental conditions.

These are my concerns. These are the stakes. Let us stop the rhetorical debate that bounds from one extreme to the other. Let us build on what is positive in the BPS approach and seek something better.

After all, no theory is completely false. The biopsychosocial model has its uses. It had a historical role, as an advance over both biological and psychoanalytic dogmatisms. But it was a temporary advance not a final solution. I am willing to allow that *some* (not all) illnesses involve biological, psychological, and social factors; examples include chronic medical conditions like diabetes and cardiovascular diseases (Engel's examples) and depressive, anxiety, and personality conditions (Grinker's focus). I am willing to grant the important of interdisciplinary work for *some* (not all) conditions; examples include psychoneuroimmunology and social epidemiology. But the BPS model, as originated by Engel and Grinker and as explicated until now by their followers, makes stronger claims. If one circumscribes the scope of these views and allows for reductionism in certain aspects of medicine and psychiatry, then one no longer subscribes to the BPS model. If one allows for prioritization of certain of these aspects (sometimes the biological should take precedence over the psychosocial or vice versa), based on empirical evidence and not simply opinion, then one no longer subscribes to the BPS model. If one wants to argue that, based on scientific evidence, clinicians should be told what to do rather than simply take whatever mix of these approaches they like, then one no longer subscribes to the BPS model.

Defenders of the biopsychosocial approach may concede on some of these specific criticisms, but they still will want to call it the BPS model. One can only conclude that human attachments to ideas learned in youth are hard to shake. Physicist Max Planck once said that scientific ideas are changed not by acceptance of rational evidence but by the passing of generations. Many mental health professionals trained in the 1980s and earlier will continue to feel allegiance to the BPS model, no matter how outdated it becomes. Those in coming generations will forget all about it. The generation coming of age today is a transitional generation, one that grew up with eclecticism as the status quo and one that left dogmatism behind long ago. Accepting what was of value in the BPS model, and then letting go of it, will happen as we mature; preparing future generations with a better overall approach to psychiatry will be a gift we can leave behind, if we have the courage to think for ourselves.

How Can We Teach It?

A Proposal for Education of Psychiatrists

It is not enough to destroy; one must build. My goal in this book is neither simply to tear down the biopsychosocial (BPS) model nor to have us return to the dogmatisms of the past. As clinicians, we all have a responsibility to move our field forward, even an inch, to show what must be done, or at least guess at it, to replace our ignorance with knowledge rather than skeptical relativism.

If the reader agrees with the content of this book, if the BPS model is to be abandoned, and a new model of medical humanism, based on Osler and Jaspers, is to replace it—if, in short, we are to take *Verstehen* seriously—how is it to be taught? How can we incorporate this approach to psychiatry and medicine into the education of doctors and psychiatrists?

Much of what I say here will apply, somewhat altered, to the education of other mental health professionals, like psychologists and social workers, but I will focus on physicians and psychiatrists for now, partly because that is my personal experience and partly because of George Engel's claim that the BPS model was mainly directed at those groups.

THE ACCREDITATION COUNCIL FOR GRADUATE MEDICAL EDUCATION REQUIREMENTS

In the United States, the Accreditation Council for Graduate Medical Education (ACGME) sets requirements for certification of residency programs for psychiatrists. (Readers can find the actual text of these requirements online at www.acgme.org.) As relevant to this book, those guidelines identify only the following among psychotherapies: "applying supportive, psychodynamic, and cognitive-behavioral psychotherapies to both brief and long-term individual practice, as well as to assuring exposure to family, couples, group and other individual evidence-based psychotherapies." The didactic curriculum is required to include the following:

(a) the major theoretical approaches to understanding the patient-doctor relationship; (b) the biological, genetic, psychological, sociocultural, economic, ethnic, gender, religious/spiritual, sexual orientation, and family factors that significantly influence physical and psychological development throughout the life cycle . . . the biological, psychological, sociocultural, and iatrogenic factors that affect the prevention, incidence, prevalence and long-term course and treatment of psychiatric disorders and . . . the history of psychiatry and its relationship to the evolution of medicine . . . [and] use of case formulation that includes neurobiological, phenomenological, psychological, and sociocultural issues involved in the management of cases.

The BPS approach is thus used to form a basis for psychiatric training. While the specific need for teaching some psychotherapies, in particular psychoanalytic views, is expressed, as is the need for research training, the only reference to any other conceptual aspect of psychiatry is the history of psychiatry. There is no mention of logic or philosophy or understanding the philosophy of science. There is no discussion of relationships between mind and brain, philosophy of mind, epistemology, or ethical theory.

Obviously, the major flaw is that conceptual topics are minimized.

TWO QUESTIONS PSYCHIATRY RESIDENCIES SHOULD ANSWER

Any program of psychiatric education, if it is conceptually sound, would have to discuss ideas beyond just pharmacology, psychoanalysis, and cognitive behavioral techniques. Some overall structure to explain those and other methods is needed. Adapting suggestions from Phillip Slavney (personal communication, January 2008), I think that a conceptually sound residency program should be so organized such that, on graduation, any psychiatric resident can answer two questions: What is psychiatry all about and what kind of psychiatrist are you? The answer to the first question is provided by method-based psychiatry. The answer to the second question is provided by choosing which methods the resident plans to apply most, and in which populations (e.g., a biological psychiatrist for bipolar disorder, or an existential psychiatrist for depression, or a psychoanalyst for the worried well).

If one were to incorporate some of the topic areas I noted as missing above, and if one wanted to specifically address some of the important thinkers and ideas I discuss in this book (in particular, a desire to teach about method-based psychiatry and a nuanced understanding of science and knowledge), a suggested curriculum might be as follows, using the *Oxford Textbook of Philosophy and Psychiatry* (OTPP) as a core text (Fulford, Thornton, and Graham 2006).

OUTLINE OF A CONCEPTUALLY ORIENTED
RESIDENCY TRAINING PROGRAM

Year I: Internship Year

Beginning six months into the year, one hour per week should be given to basic conceptual discussions of medicine and psychiatry. Residents will completely read William Osler's *Aequenimitas* (Osler 1948) as a basic text. Sections of the *OTPP* on phenomenology and philosophy of science will be read.

Year II: Inpatient Year

For one hour weekly, residents will read and discuss George Engel's classic papers, Roy Grinker Sr.'s writings, and Paul McHugh and Phillip Slavney's *Perspectives of Psychiatry*. Sections of the *OTPP* on diagnostic classification and epistemology will be read.

Year III: Outpatient Year

For one hour weekly, residents will read and discuss Leston Havens's *Approaches to the Mind,* and selections from Emil Kraepelin, Phillippe Pinel, Adolf Meyer, and Aubrey Lewis, among others. Selections of the *OTPP* on philosophy of mind will be read. Residents will also read selected poems related to medicine and psychiatry.

Year IV: Advanced Training Year

Too many residents suffer from senioritis, feeling they know all there is to know. A rude awakening awaits them in real-world clinical practice, if, as is often the case, they take it easy in this largely elective year, or, even worse, if they forgo it entirely in conjunction with other training (most commonly combining this last year of adult psychiatry training with the first year of child psychiatry fellowship).

This final year is the most important year in psychiatric training, where the broad but superficial education of prior years can be deepened and made profound. Now residents could be capable of more difficult and detailed readings in conceptual psychiatry. One approach would be as follows: For one hour weekly, residents will read and discuss selections from Karl Jaspers's *General Psychopathology* and selected contemporary papers on philosophy and psychiatry. Sections of the *OTPP* on Jaspers and on ethics will be read. Residents will also read and discuss selected poems and literary essays about medicine and psychiatry.

A CONCEPTUAL STRUCTURE FOR RESIDENCY TRAINING

McHugh and Slavney published, in the *Oxford Textbook of Psychiatry* (Fulford, Thornton, and Graham 2006), their outline for the education of psychiatrists, much of which agrees with my critique above. They hold that psychiatric education should have a conceptual structure, based on their perspectives of psychiatry. I do not disagree with their approach, though I would suggest that the method-based psychiatry model, more broadly conceived, should be that structure. This would include their perspectives approach but also involve study of Havens's four schools taxonomy and Jaspers's *Verstehen/ Erklären* demarcation. Nor would my conceptual structure be limited to these method-based models: the roots of these different views would need to be studied, leading to broader exposure to philosophy (such as the philosophy of pragmatism, philosophy of science, mind-brain theories), and other nondogmatic noneclectic views (such as "integrationism" as in the work of Eric Kandel). I firmly agree with McHugh and Slavney, though, that the biggest flaw in psychiatric education today is the absence of a "coherent conceptual structure," and I would add that the source of this flaw is in the widespread acceptance of BPS eclecticism, driven by our postmodernist intuitions. We do not need to back to dogmatism, however: we have good alternatives, a method-based psychiatry that is more conceptually sound than evidence-based medicine and more scientific than either dogmatism or BPS eclecticism.

OBJECTIONS

Some will be skeptical about this proposal. The specific content of teaching suggested here is obviously open to change. The point is to cover the subject areas of philosophy and conceptual aspects of psychiatry, as well as provide exposure to the humanities in medicine.

Skeptics also might agree with Aubrey Lewis, the leader of twentieth-century British psychiatry, who once wrote in an article about the education of psychiatrists:

> You may be disposed to quarrel with my frequent use of the word "training," as though a psychiatrist were an athlete or a circus elephant. . . . By the time a man enters on the postgraduate study of psychiatry, his general education should be able to look after itself and should gain from all his experience: if it cannot, the horse is out, and it will be idle to close the stable door by formal teaching. . . . The whole of the psychiatrist's postgraduate studies should train him in reasoning and understanding. . . . And surely example and steady guidance, rather than precepts and "a course," are the best corrective for defects in that general education which should fit a man to combine the scientific and the humane temper in his studies, as the psychiatrist needs to. (Lewis 1967, p. 80)

I do not share Lewis's pessimism. Given the sorry state of American education in the humanities (all the way from elementary to high school to university to medical school), typical psychiatric residents need specific attention, and sustained effort, to augment their conceptual and humanistic knowledge, if we are to take seriously the notion that psychiatry should be neither dogmatic nor eclectic.

Otherwise, we would have to rely, as we have to date, on the self-motivation of residents to pursue these topics. And, though the best teaching is self-motivated, students and residents can learn, even if their motivation is limited, when exposed sufficiently to different ideas or approaches. The key is that educators need to value those ideas and make them a central part of the curriculum. It is clear, in my view, that psychoanalytic teaching is much more detailed in many programs than it needs to be for contemporary practice; the same could be said about biological teaching in other programs. Some room needs to be made for the bigger picture, not to take away from these other parts of psychiatry, but to provide the larger context without which they are at best a source of confusion and at worst a cause for dogmatism.

Interested residents could be directed by faculty to independent reading, and it is hoped that this conceptual base not only would produce a more intellectually sound profession but also it will create practitioners who are not averse to thinking and who have a solid basis for continuing to think critically and conceptually throughout their careers.

Our medical students and psychiatric residents are capable of appreciating much more than we bother to teach them. It is time we worked their minds and not just their capacities to emulate and regurgitate. Wilhelm Dilthey would have known they were capable of it, for, after all: "We always understand more than we know" (Ermarth 1978, p. 251).

Notes

CHAPTER ONE: The Perils of Open-mindedness

1. In this perspective, Meyer was ahead of his time. He applied the public health perspective to disease long before most other leading psychiatrists considered it. One of his students, Aubrey Lewis, led the British school of psychiatry centered around the Maudsley Hospital at the University of London; with his student Michael Shepherd, Lewis brought public health and epidemiology into psychiatry as a key means of understanding mental illness. In their efforts, they were following in the tradition of Meyer.

2. Meyer recommended teeth extraction, almost as an afterthought, in addition to self-help techniques and generally supportive psychotherapy, to a prominent Canadian politician, MacKenzie King, who came to the Johns Hopkins Hospital to be treated for various psychosomatic ailments as well as some clear psychopathology (probably auditory hallucinations) in the late 1910s (before King became famous as Canada's prime minister in the 1920s). King was impressed by Meyer's supportive manner, and it seems that Meyer focused on psychological support as the key to King's treatment, but he also added Cotton's method of teeth extraction, just in case (Roazen 1993a).

3. Worldwide about fifty thousand lobotomies had been performed by the time the Nobel was awarded for it in 1949. After World War II, while lobotomy was highly common in the West, it was banned in West Germany and in the Soviet Union. The 1949 Nobel Prize spurred interest in the practice. Freeman himself had nominated Antonio Caetano de Abreu Freire Egas Moniz for the Nobel Prize for Medicine and was somewhat influential in the campaign that led to his receiving the award. It is ironic that in that same year, Australian psychiatrist John Cade would discover lithium, an effective treatment that to this day continues to be probably the most effective psychotropic medication ever; yet after the Moniz fiasco, the Nobel committee shied away from giving awards for direct treatment of mental illness, and thus the clinical discoverers of lithium, antipsychotics, and antidepressants have never been duly recognized.

CHAPTER TWO: So Many Theories, So Little Time

1. The only overall "rapprochement" that Williams saw was, as we will see with both Roy Grinker Sr. and George Engel, a reliance on the holistic theories derived from general systems theory (Williams cites the founder of that theory, Ludwig von Bertalanffy).

2. Outside of psychiatry and psychology, warnings about eclecticism have also been made. For instance, in nursing, it has been suggested that the field is "drowning in eclecticism": "A seemingly unlimited range of theories from multiple disciplines (about

a seemingly unlimited range of phenomena) are used throughout the professional practice and scholarship of nurses. . . . Eclecticism—defined as selecting the best or more favored from various sources, styles, or methods—is not, in and of itself, a 'bad' thing" (Cody 1996). But it is a problem in nursing when it consists of "constantly borrowing" from other disciplines rather than "growing the body of knowledge that is nursing's own." There is a "miasma of endless, unbridled theory sampling." Hence "nurses find themselves in effect simmering in a theoretical soup." This results in "the 'black bag' approach to selection and application of theories . . . as the modus operandi of many practicing nurses and scholars." "To maintain in that grab bag a collection of theories for use that are philosophically and logically incompatible with one another is intellectually and ethically indefensible." The consequences are that "the enforced eclecticism in contemporary nursing reduces the performing art of nursing to imitation and pastiche" (Cody 1996). Clearly, eclecticism can get, and perhaps has gotten, out of hand, not only in psychiatry but in allied disciplines such as nursing.

3. This approach, which has Kantian roots in philosophy of mind, was similarly expressed by Karl Jaspers years earlier (though unreferenced by Yager).

4. This definition is similar to Karl Jaspers's methodological consciousness, or the pluralistic model I proposed in *The Concepts of Psychiatry* (Johns Hopkins University Press, 2003).

5. Ibid.

6. Ibid.

CHAPTER THREE: Riding Madly in All Directions

1. Sigmund Freud stated that his usual fee was $25 per hour and that even in his old age he was obliged to continue seeing patients and charging such fees to make a living. Roy Grinker apparently expressed a concern about being able to provide such funds, leading Freud to describe a sliding scale that he could provide as an exception, with no lower than $10 per hour. Freud's higher rate translates to about $400 per hour today (using a 1933 inflation conversion factor of 0.065, http//oregonstate.edu/dept/pol-sci/fac/sahr/sahr.htm), and the lower rate to somewhat less than $200 per hour. I have known some senior psychoanalysts and other therapists that charge in Freud's range; perhaps there should be a rule that no psychotherapist should be allowed to charge more than the greatest psychoanalyst who ever lived! The slightly unseemly bickering over fees ended in Freud's ultimate acceptance of Grinker as a patient. It appears that Grinker initially planned to see Sandor Ferenczi in Budapest, perhaps due to lower fees, but switched to Freud after Ferenczi died unexpectedly.

2. In numerous articles and books from the 1950s to the 1970s, Grinker makes the point that eclecticism in psychiatry largely grew out of a reaction to Freudian orthodoxy. Grinker is always careful to praise Freud himself and the "early pioneers" who "flew by the seat of their pants." He emphasized how Freud, besides the obvious fact of emphasizing psychological concepts for neuroses, also utilized both biological concepts (like the death instinct) and social concepts (as in Freud's paper "Group Psychology and the Analysis of the Ego"). Yet after Freud, the biological and social aspects of illness were extruded from orthodox psychoanalysis, leading to heterodoxies that emphasized them (such as Karen Horney and Harry Stack Sullivan for social aspects and

Melanie Klein for biological concepts). Eclecticism in psychoanalysis, Grinker emphasized, meant being open to biological and social concepts, as opposed to just individual psychology. Grinker clearly saw a biopsychosocial (BPS) approach to psychiatry as
a savior of psychoanalysis. In 1966, he described how psychoanalysis had started as an
"open-system," with a great deal of creativity and experimentation among the early pioneers; later it became a "closed-system libido" ideology (Grinker 1966). The BPS approach would allow it to be part of an "open-system psychiatry" again, thus reviving
psychoanalysis as an "open-system adaptational" theory (p. 121). It was not a competing approach but rather a perspective than could be used "without sacrificing any of
the dynamic concepts of psychoanalysis" (p. 116).

3. Earlier than either Grinker or Engel, without using the BPS label, perhaps the
first description of the basic idea needs to be attributed to John Romano and Engel in
1947, who wrote in an article of the need for a "more comprehensive frame of reference
or conceptual scheme of disease [than that] with which the student had heretofore
been . . . familiar . . . [a] conceptual scheme . . . in which psychological and social facts
exist or coexist with more impersonal biological factors, eventually to cause, provoke,
or otherwise modify variations in the total human biological behavior" (Brown 2003,
204). Also Victor Frankl's 1946 book, *The Doctor and the Soul,* refers to humanity as
a "somatopsychospiritual" entity. Frankl partly wrote his manuscript before being im-
prisoned in Nazi concentration camps from 1942 to 1945. After his survival and release,
he completed his work with the above formulation as the basis for his existential psychotherapy (he called it "logotherapy"; Frankl 1986). Thus, perhaps we should credit
Frankl for first formulating the BPS concept, Romano next, and then Grinker for most
clearly expounding on it. Engel was not its sole creator by any means.

4. Historian Edward Shorter, distinctly underwhelmed by the intellectual power of
the BPS model, points out that much of the impact of the model may simply come
from the catchy phrase, or memorable label, rather than any special content (Shorter
2005).

CHAPTER FOUR: A New Model of Medicine

1. Engel's publications involved some very *unbiopsychosocial* titles: G. L. Engel,
I. Chao, The comparative distribution of organic phosphorus compounds in the cardiac and striated muscles of limulus polyphemus, *Journal of Biological Chemistry* 108
(1935): 389–93; G. L. Engel, R. W. Gerard, The phosphorus metabolism of invertebrate
nerve, *Journal of Biological Chemistry* 112 (1935): 379–92.

2. One might view the BPS model as a good one for ulcerative colitis without seeing special relevance to manic-depressive illness.

3. The paper is not particularly impressive. It basically consists of a rejection of
single etiology theories of disease and a statement of the holistic approach to health
and disease that directly seemed like a translation (though unattributed) from general
systems theory. There is a discussion of the importance of psychological stress in biological factors in illness, with allusions to social factors, but the three aspects are not
formally united in a model of illness. Engel does, however, make some points that turn
out to be important in understanding the basis of his later model. They include the following:

a.   He is opposed to the notion that health can be clearly demarcated from disease.

b.   He is opposed to the view that disease consists of something one *has,* as in the germ theory, that simply enters one's body and is foreign to it. Disease is rather always a complex interaction between the body and the environment.

c.   Biological reductionism asks only "how" questions about the nature of disease but not "why." For instance, peptic ulcer involves excessive vagal nerve activity, but why that happens (presumably the role of psychological stress) is ignored.

d.   Regarding nosology, diagnostic labels are not necessarily bad in themselves but they can be inhibitory instead of helpful. When our knowledge of a condition is limited, the labels are only general approximations; they change, and should change, as our knowledge improves. But if they are taken as correct and complete when they merely reflect such immature knowledge, they can inhibit more investigation. Also, "a diagnostic label rarely, if ever, fully defines the illness" (p. 463). Thus, unlike psychoanalysts, Engel viewed diagnosis as often necessary, but unlike Kraepelinians, he did not view it as sufficient for the clinical understanding of illness: "Clinical diagnosis . . . is not an end in itself" (p. 464).

e.   He admits that health is difficult to define (p. 470).

f.   In the key part of the paper on the "necessary and sufficient conditions" for disease, he describes that "one never deals with a single etiologic factor in the genesis of a disease state, although one factor may be more important than others, or there may be practical advantages in paying more attention to one factor than to others. . . . The scientific approach to disease assumes multiple factors, some more proximate, some more distant in time; some more specific, some more general in their effects; some necessary, but not in themselves sufficient to bring about the disease" (pp. 473–74).

g.   He then identifies the factors involved in the etiology of disease: genetic, developmental, and "factors that strain the current capacities of the organism." Among the last of these factors are those that "injure by virtue of physical and/or chemical properties," other physical factors, "microorganisms and parasites," and "psychological stress."

h.   He finally lays the most emphasis on psychological stress, which he subdivides as "loss or threat of loss of psychic objects," "injury to the body . . . actual or threatened" leading to psychological stress, and "frustration of drives." *Note the strong psychoanalytic imagery.*

i.   He also describes how patterns of response to stress are also "factors in determining the manifestations of illness" (p. 483).

j.   He concludes (p. 485): "No linear concept of etiology is appropriate; rather, the pathogenesis of disease involves a series of negative and positive feedbacks with multiple simultaneous and sequential changes potentially affecting any system of the body. The central nervous system is so organized functionally that a reciprocal interrelationship between the mental apparatus and the rest of the body in the pathogenesis of disease states and maintenance of health is not only possible but inevitable."

4. It might be argued that it is not factually correct for us to view the modern BPS model in psychiatry as primarily the handiwork of George Engel. After all, as discussed above, Engel was primarily interested in changing the face of general medicine, not just psychiatry. An anonymous critic in *Perspectives in Biology in Medicine* who reviewed some of my writing, now in the text here, had the following reaction:

> Much if not all criticism that the author formulates with respect to the BPS seems misdirected, since what Engel articulated at the time is merely that medical phenomena are complex and their understanding requires incorporation of diverse material (e.g., ideas, techniques, social and cultural background, neurobiology, general biology etc) instead of evolving in a reductionist pathway. The article in *Science* buttressed its construal of medical phenomena in a far broader context than the author acknowledges, so as to include general biology, culture, society, and biomedical insights; and it decried and/or warned against the drift toward biological reductionism. It was as a broadly based general physician/scientist/educator that he spoke and not as a psychoanalyst! . . . Furthermore, Engel's paper for psychiatrists was partly a political statement. The establishment figures who invited him and then could use his ideas for their own purposes were the beneficiaries. It is true that much was made of BPS for psychiatry at the time, but by others. Engel was suspect about psychiatry and his identity was hardly that of a psychiatrist but as a general physician, educator, and thinker in medicine interested in a broad conception of disease. However, Engel's BPS became reified as an "important," new path breaking and scientifically compelling "model" . . . Although termed a model, Engel's article was really a generally, all encompassing, theoretical point of view, rather than a model to be used to order thought and methodology in a specific empirical way. Rather than . . . criticizing the BPS, criticism should be directed at those who extolled BPS in the first place, making more of Engel's ideas than he proposed, or intended to propose, and than his ideas really entailed. Those who championed BPS as a credible theoretical articulation about and for scientific, research, and clinical matters . . . can be argued to have reflected a naïve, simplistic view of psychiatry and medicine (that something as complex as disease or psychiatric conditions, and ways to deal with these in a scientifically and clinically satisfactory manner, can be formulated as and reduced to a simple model for all aspects of its understanding) . . . . Rather, the focus should be on the BPS as a general and political document, even a manifesto of sorts, of a senior, respected, influential, humane, thinker/clinician/educator/researcher concerned about the direction medicine was taking. This document was then misinterpreted, misappropriated, and exploited as either a set of ideas the implications of which were misunderstood and exaggerated or as helpful in the pursuit of political agendas Engel had not contemplated and certainly did not appear to intend.

This critic accepts the negative consequences of the BPS model while seeking to protect the value and integrity of the work of Engel himself. I have no doubt that Engel as a man was a wonderful person and that his intentions were anything but the best, but one cannot avoid the fact that intellectuals have a heavy responsibility: ideas have consequences. Anyone engaged in intellectual work has to take responsibility for his ideas and partly also to whatever uses those ideas are given by others. This is because others see aspects of one's ideas that they can exploit for those other purposes. The ideas have to be vulnerable to such use, and it is this vulnerability for which the original thinker needs to take responsibility. Thus, Marx cannot be fully exonerated for the excesses of Lenin or Stalin, even though he was also interpreted in much more humane ways by Eduard Bernstein and Karl Kautsky. Similarly, Freud is partly responsible for all varieties of psychoanalysis, even though he fully adhered to only his own formulation. Marx famously said, in French for effect: "Moi, je ne suis pas Marxiste" (Me, I am not a Marxist) to distance himself from some who used his ideas. Indeed, despite all the excesses of later communism, Marx the man and thinker has great merit. So too with Engel; he has great merit, but this need not exonerate us from looking to the reasons why his theory was able to be used in ways that may have proved harmful to psychiatry.

CHAPTER FIVE: Before and After

1. Note the Meyerian language: "failures of the organism to adjust . . . to changes in the environment."

2. The nonprofit corporation is called "OneHealth." The event was funded by a pharmaceutical company, Novartis, which raises questions about whether the pharmaceutical industry sees the BPS model as being to its benefit (see chapter 9).

3. In 1989, as a medical student, I was perhaps one of the few who crossed that street, attending a neurology rotation at King's College and informally going to seminars and meetings at Maudsley Hospital.

4. Malmgren expanded on this in the discussion (pp. 36–37): "I said it doesn't make sense to talk about a psychological process and its underlying substrate interacting, because then you are in a sense talking about the same thing twice (although in different ways). It is like saying that the floor is clean because I have used a vacuum cleaner *and* have used an electric machine that works by sucking air. You cannot look at these as partial causes, because the vacuum cleaning process is supervenient on the workings of the electric machine and suction pump. One could express the same point by saying that since the electric machine is the physical realization of a vacuum cleaner, they are not really two things."

CHAPTER SIX: Cease-fire

1. It is difficult to give a single reference for this brief history of Boston psychiatry. I have learned it firsthand through personal communications over the years with the following persons among others: Ross Baldessarini, a student of Kety; Leston Havens, a student of Semrad; and Jacob Katzow, who trained at Mass Mental in the 1960s and was a friend of Klerman. Some of this history can also be found in recollections of persons such as Eric Kandel (1998).

2. Joseph P. Kennedy once remarked that he would sell voters on his son, John F. Kennedy, like people sell soap flakes.

3. Psychiatric historian Edward Shorter first examined the roots of the BPS model in Engel's work. Shorter noted that Engel's thinking along these lines dates to the early 1950s (though he did not acknowledge the important influence of Grinker in advancing the model as well). Shorter argued that the BPS model failed to achieve more influence due to the success of psychopharmacology. After Engel, he argued, the BPS

model was used by psychotherapy-oriented clinicians to fight the medication approach to psychiatry; it would lead, in effect, to "an inrush of psychoanalysis through the back door, to fuzzy-ize [the] profession again." After all the years of effort to defeat psychoanalytic dogmatism, the biological leaders of American psychiatry were wary of such a potential Trojan horse (Shorter 2005).

CHAPTER SEVEN: Drowning in Data

1. One might have hoped for some guidance on how the BPS model can help research from specific articles written in honor of Engel, such as in the 1980 retirement Festschrift organized by his University of Rochester colleagues (published as a supplement of the journal *Psychosomatic Medicine*). The title of one article certainly seems promising: "Implications of the biopsychosocial model for research in psychiatry" (Reiser 1980). Yet the article's main idea seems to be that the BPS model can provide a general rationale for avoiding reductionism, to know that everything is interrelated. While this kind of meta-theory, as Grinker put it, may be generally useful in some ways, it does not seem to have direct utility for research. In fact, rather than providing any details about how this approach can be applied in research, the article consists of four clinical cases of the proposed clinical uses of the model.

In a qualitative study of the views of Engel's former students, it was clear that the BPS model was not easy to integrate with research. They wrote about tensions between practicing the BPS approach and "doing formal research." As one put it, "For me it was finally coming to realize that I don't have to be doing formal research in order to be scientific about what I'm about with patients; to be an Engelite and not to be doing that, was a source of tension for me for a number of years" (Dombeck et al. 2003, p. 249). Most of Engel's followers did *not* become successful clinical researchers. The example of one exception is informative: "Another former fellow . . . was determined that the only way for him to be successful in his practice of the approach was to also succeed in doing formal research. This former fellow was well established away from Rochester. He was interviewed by telephone: 'I wrote a lot of grants and got rejected, and in asking why I was rejected, one editor said, it is hard to convince those who won't be convinced. From that, I worked to reshape the Biopsychosocial Model in a way that people could understand it. I started getting funded and [to] write. . . . Research needs to be done in the mainstream. . . . Perhaps George Engel was the Messiah and I was the Apostle. I had another mentor, Dr. ____, who helped me play the game in the mainstream. . . . Societal pressures were moving us away from the model. . . . The problem is how to handle being different with the help of your mentor. I was fully convinced I was right, but I needed mentors. As I got established I felt different, but not undervalued" (Dombeck et al. 2003).

CHAPTER EIGHT: Teaching Eclecticism

1. Engel then gives a case example of a patient who had to receive an arterial puncture, got anxious, and then developed a ventricular fibrillation. To view this case as nothing more than the biological fact of ventricular fibrillation, without assessing the preceding anxiety and the painful experience of arterial puncture, would seem inadequate. This case would seem to be, in a sense, a clear example of needing to pay atten-

tion to the interplay of psychological and biological states. In the context of general medicine, where Engel was focused, it seems reasonable, but its relevance in cases of psychiatric illness was never directly expanded on by Engel.

2. Here is another example of the limitations of the BPS model for medical students. One author described a medical student who had strong intuitive capacities in relationships and interviewing skills that would have indicated great skill in psychiatry. Yet the author could not convince the student to consider psychiatric residency as opposed to going into other medical specialties: "I need something to hand my hat on," the student said. "I'm interested in psychiatry and would go into it, but I'm not interested in a field that is based primarily on hunch and intuition" (Eaton 1980). The author goes on to note that "we have abandoned our medically students intellectually by not providing them conceptual frameworks" for their intuitive skills in psychiatry, but that the BPS model now provides that "conceptual base" and "philosophic home." As noted above, however, these hopes have not been fulfilled. Psychiatry seems as confusing as ever to medical students, and the BPS model has not helped to clarify matters and clearly has not translated into increasing psychiatric specialization by U.S. medical students.

CHAPTER NINE: Psychopharmacology Awry

1. See S. N. Ghaemi, *The Concepts of Psychiatry* (Johns Hopkins University Press, 2003).

2. See S. N. Ghaemi (Editor), *Polypharmacy in Psychiatry* (New York: Marcel Dekker, 2002).

CHAPTER TEN: The Vagaries of the Real World

1. A particularly influential paper in the United Kingdom rephrased this movement in the concept of "postpsychiatry" (Bracken and Thomas 2001), with a consequent rise in a group of psychiatrists formed around a "Critical Psychiatry" website (www.critpsy net.freeuk.com). A recent book seeks to extend this perspective to American psychiatry (Lewis 2006).

2. This oversimplified version of the "medical model" is not William Osler's medical model.

3. www.mentalhealthcommission.gov.

CHAPTER TWELVE: Osler's Ghost

1. It is perhaps coincidental that Engel spent a summer as a medical student, on the advice of his uncle, doing countless autopsies. Engel later rebelled against this classic Oslerian education.

2. There used to be a time when every medical student received Osler's selected essays entitled *Aequenimitas* (Osler 1948) on graduating from medical school (sometimes courtesy of pharmaceutical companies). Modern medicine would be more improved if this tradition were restored than if the technology of MRIs and PET scanning were to be improved a hundredfold.

3. This definition comes from Charles Odegaard (1986).

4. Medical historian Theodore Brown, of the University of Rochester.

5. *Moriturum te salutamus* means "We who are about to die, salute you!" This was the motto of the gladiators, spoken to Caesar, before they began a fight.

CHAPTER THIRTEEN: The Two Cultures

1. This is not to say that all physicians are averse to the humanities. Indeed there is a rich tradition of physician-writers and even anthologies of poetry written by physicians, such as the weekly poems of *JAMA* (Breedlove 1998). Despite this tradition, however, most physicians, including psychiatrists, are more averse to the humanities than most nonphysicians are.

2. Some might say that I am setting up a straw man: Which physician would say that an appreciation of the "humanity" or individuality of her patients would interfere with her medical abilities? This is not a straw man: I am responding to Engel's claim that anyone who rejects the BPS model would have to be biological reductionist, ignoring the human component of medicine. My claim is that Engel is wrong: that a good case can be made that biological approaches to medicine are enhanced by humanism, and thus we do not need to turn to the BPS model instead. My straw man is made of flesh and blood: George Engel.

3. Perhaps the main philosophical work on this topic is that of George Lakoff, who argued that metaphor is at the basis of all language and all thought. Lakoff suggested that it was less relevant to physical science, consistent with William Dilthey's distinctions (see chapter 14; Lakoff and Johnson 1980).

4. I might be asked why I focus on poetry and do not give equal time to literature, theater, religion, history, classics, sports, fashion, and popular culture, which might be viewed as more important aids for connecting with a patient. I would support all these perspectives, but the root of all the humanities has to do with stories and metaphor, for which we have the most sources, dating back millennia, in literature and poetry.

5. I realize that linguistics is a large and complex field, that this statement has not been proven here, and that other views are held by experts. I will not defend it here, nor is it central to my thesis about the importance of poetry and the humanities to human knowledge in general and to medicine in particular. Yet, some linguistic theorists, like Lakoff, do hold this view.

6. I thank Ronald Pies for showing me this wonderful poem by Williams and making this key connection.

7. There is more to this conflict between the two cultures: Dilthey talks about two cognitive processes or ways of knowing (see next chapter).

8. Engel felt psychoanalysis did the latter job better than poetry; perhaps, despite his ample borrowing from Goethe and Shakespeare and his classical education, Freud would have agreed. If we were forced to choose, however, between destroying all of Engel's, or even Freud's, works and keeping those of Goethe or Shakespeare or Homer, or vice versa, the decision is clear.

CHAPTER FOURTEEN: Between Science and the Humanities

1. Ralph Waldo Emerson once wrote that great philosophers eventually become so ingrained in a culture that we carry around their ideas in our bones; we think their

thoughts without knowing where they came from. This is the case with the postmodernist relativism that can be traced to Michel Foucault and other French philosophers of the 1960s.

2. The distinction was first made by German philosopher of history J. G. Droysen in 1858, where he actually identified three kinds of knowledge: "the philosophical method, the physical method, and the historical method." The aims of the three methods were seen by Droysen as to know (*Erkennen*), to explain (*Erklären*), and to understand (*Verstehen;* Von Wright 1971). It is interesting how the rational form of knowledge (*Erkennen*) has become intertwined now with the more empirical experience-based knowledge of *Erklären*.

3. As one commentator puts it: "Human beings think, feel, and aspire; they have a point of view of their own, which we need to appreciate if we are to make sense of their behavior. This is what Dilthey's theory of understanding is about" (p. 52, Rickman).

4. Once, when I tried to introduce a course at Harvard Medical School on Jaspers's ideas, the rejection of my proposal was accompanied by a critique wondering why we should be wasting our lecture time on long-dead German professors. I suspect that some of my readers may have a similar reaction at this point. I may have succeeded in destroying their faith in the BPS model; but what have I given them in its place? Two German words! How disappointing. In a classic history of ideas, American intellectual H. Stuart Hughes once called *Verstehen* "the most difficult problem that I have confronted in the present study—the murkiest of the dark corners in the labyrinth of German social science methods" (Rickman 1988, p. 176). I hope my presentation is somewhat clarifying, however (with more explanation will be found in chapter 15). Thus I must ask my readers to grant me one concession: though I speak and write in English, work in the United States, and have rejected some proudly American thinkers in Grinker and Engel, this does not make the foreign names of Dilthey and Jaspers and the strange jargon of *Verstehen* and *Erklären* thereby inferior.

5. Dilthey himself emphasized, putting it in his own language, this triad of features as *Verstehen*: first, getting into the "lived experience" (*Erlebnis*) of another person: second, understanding the verbal and nonverbal expressions of another person; and third, the creation of a synthetic meaning from the whole.

6. By the science of psychology, Engel mostly meant psychoanalysis: the claim that psychoanalysis is a science, based on *Erklären*, like biological sciences, can be true only in an alternate universe.

7. Slavney explained to me that he and McHugh perhaps were not explicit about the relevance of the humanities, especially in the life story perspective, because they saw it as self-evident. McHugh wrote thus in "Another psychiatrist's Shakespeare" (McHugh 2006): "Shakespeare is our contemporary. He deals with so much and even shows us psychiatrists how we might function with understanding. In his realism Shakespeare offers not an 'essence' of humankind, a single vision of our minds, but a multiplicity of visions, each of which carries a message for reflections."

CHAPTER FIFTEEN: The Meaning of Meaning

1. *Geisteswissenschaften.* The phrase was originally coined in 1863 as a way to translate from English into German John Stuart Mill's term "the moral sciences," which he was contrasting to "the physical sciences." Dilthey then expanded and popularized the

German term (Von Wright 1971). One could limit the term to social sciences, like sociology and anthropology, or scientific studies of human behavior, thus including psychology. One group of thinkers (led by Heinrich Rickert) contemporaneous to Dilthey did so, and they preferred the term *Kulturwissenschaften* (cultural sciences). Dilthey gave much thought to this topic and wanted to include what are not generally considered "sciences," namely, poetry and art and literature, and thus he kept the broader term *human sciences*. Because literature would not seem to be a science in the same sense as these other disciplines, some have suggested the term "human studies." I have decided to go with the latter, because in English "human sciences" is too narrow.

2. I use the term *synthetic meaning* to get across how Dilthey saw this final act as pulling together everything else and providing a general concept or theory that would make sense of the overall human phenomenon being studied; Dilthey simply used the word *Verstehen* for this third phase, but since the whole process is usually identified with *Verstehen*, I will use the term "synthetic meaning." Another way of putting together the various aspects of *Verstehen* as described by Dilthey is to follow five parts, as described by Wiggins and Schwartz: (1) *Einfuhlen*, or empathy; (2) *Mitfuhlen*, or sympathy; (3) *Nachenleben*, or re-experiencing; (4) *Nachleben*, or reliving; and (5) *Nachbilden*, or re-creating (Wiggins and Schwartz 1997). One gets the sense of the psychological richness implied by Dilthey's concept of *Verstehen* in these five components. Finally, it should be noted that Dilthey's *Verstehen* was not a purely cognitive or psychological construct; it was not just something that we think rationally or even that we feel with our emotions. For Dilthey, *Verstehen* was the result of our entire being—using not only our intellect and our emotions but also our souls, our bodies, our culture, our history—all aspects of our being are relevant to *Verstehen* (R. Makkreel, personal communication, March 2008). This is one important reason why literature and poetry also mattered to Dilthey as part of the process of *Verstehen*.

3. Makkreel writes: "In his general discussion of the human studies, Dilthey had denied that they dealt with objects (*Objekten*) different in kind from those of the natural sciences. Yet in indicating that a mere methodological distinction is not enough, he now claims that there is a difference in the subject matter of history due to an exclusive attention to the significance of its data" (Makkreel 1992, p. 306).

CHAPTER SIXTEEN: The Beginning of a Solution

1. I quoted that parable in detail in *The Concepts of Psychiatry* (Johns Hopkins University Press, 2003).

2. I have interpreted Kety's parable in a pluralistic way, which I derive from a separate tradition in psychiatry, one not derived from the two dogmas of Kraepelin and Freud but rather from the profound method-based psychiatry of Karl Jaspers (see *The Concepts of Psychiatry*).

3. See *The Concepts of Psychiatry*.

4. The historical genealogy in psychiatry, as opposed to philosophy, of the evolution of Jaspers's views is follows: The psychologically trained Kraepelin and the neurologically trained Freud were criticized and synthesized by the methodological Jaspers. Jaspers trained in the Heidelberg department right after the period of Emil Kraepelin's chairmanship there, so it was heavily still influenced by Kraepelin's model under his successor Franz Nissl, a neuroanatomically oriented psychiatrist. One of Jaspers's stu-

dents was Willy Mayer-Gross, who left during the Nazi era and went to the United Kingdom. Most Freudians went to the United States. Hence, the United States became heavily psychoanalytic, and the United Kingdom became more Jaspersian. The eventual twentieth-century leader of British psychiatry, Aubrey Lewis, had trained for a time with Adolf Meyer and was also influenced by Mayer-Gross. Thus, British psychiatry, as led by Lewis at the Maudsley Hospital, became a Meyerian-Jaspersian amalgamation. Meanwhile, American psychiatry produced Harry Stack Sullivan, who reinterpreted Freudian notions with more of an interpersonal orientation. Sullivanian views, mixed with Freud and existential notions, influenced the key teacher of Harvard psychiatrists Elvin Semrad. Semrad was the mentor of Leston Havens. As a medical student, Paul McHugh was mentored by Havens and exposed to Semrad, as well as Mandel Cohen, a Harvard psychiatrist previously trained by Meyer. McHugh later trained Phillip Slavney and others influential in the development of philosophy and psychiatry, such as Michael Schwartz and Marshal Folstein. As a medical student, I met McHugh and Havens when I interviewed in their programs at the Johns Hopkins Hospital and Cambridge Hospital, respectively. I studied under Havens during a medical student rotation and observed McHugh in case conferences when I visited Hopkins on occasion. After moving to Boston for my Harvard residency at McLean Hospital, many of my supervisors were former students of Semrad. Among them, Walker Shields introduced me to the Tavistock approach to psychoanalytic thinking and Alfred Marguelis conducted a reading seminar with me on his book about empathy (Marguelis 1989). Later, when I joined the Cambridge faculty for five years, I had weekly supervision with Havens. I continued to interact with McHugh at conferences and symposia over the past decade.

CHAPTER SEVENTEEN: A New Psychiatric Humanism

1. The contributions of Jaspers can be found in *General Psychopathology* in chapter 12 ("Nosology: The Synthesis of Disease Entities") and the last two chapters of this book (Part 6, "The Human Being as a Whole;" chapter 4: "The Concept of Health and Illness"; chapter 5: "The Meaning of Medical Practice").

2. All following quotations by Lewis in this section refer to this source. The original article was titled "Health as a Social Concept."

Afterword

1. A claim made in the 2008 presidential election by Republican candidate John McCain.

2. See my full critique of Healy's social constructionist history of bipolar disorder at Metapsychology Online: *A Short History of Bipolar Disorder,* by David Healy, published by Johns Hopkins University Press, 2008. Review by S. Nassir Ghaemi, MD, MA, MPH vol. 12, no. 40 (September 30, 2008) at http://metapsychology.mentalhelp.net/.

A Brief Glossary of Concepts

I hope that this glossary assists readers in understanding my use of certain terms in this book. These definitions are not meant to be exhaustive but may provide some shorthand as readers seek to understand these concepts that are more fully spelled out in the text. Also please note that words are defined as they apply in this book, not with the meanings that might be more commonly used. I have left nuances out for the sake of brevity. Again, readers should read these comments only as markers, signposts, not complete definitions, for which they should turn to the text itself.

Biopsychosocial model: This whole book is the definition of this model. But a brief starting point definition might be the notion that all illness has biological, psychological, and social aspects. Varying further interpretations from this starting point can be found in the work of George Engel and Roy Grinker and others, as further described in the text. Contrast with *medical humanism.* See its role in psychiatry in *eclecticism.*

Dogmatism: The view that a single method or theory explains all, or most, of psychiatry.

Eclecticism: A model that views any theory or method as potentially correct, but no theory or method as definitively incorrect. More is better. All theories should be used together. The choice of method is based on doctor or patient preference or values. In political analogy: anarchism. See contrast with *pluralism* and *method-based psychiatry.*

Erklären: Causal explanation. The method of empirical science, identifying causes and effects in the real world of experience. An objective, third-person perspective. Associated with statistics and biological experimentation in psychiatry. Attends to general, not unique, aspects of phenomena. Contrasts with *Verstehen.*

Evidence-based medicine: For the purposes of this book, the view that *Erklären*-based positivistic science can produce truth. Basically, an instantiation of biological dogmatism. Contrasts with *method-based psychiatry.*

General systems theory: A philosophy of biology used by proponents of the biopsychosocial model as a means to provide conceptual grounding, so as to avoid "anything goes" eclecticism. General systems theory argues that an organism can be understood only as a complex of a multiple systems not at any one level of those systems (i.e., not just at the molecular level but through appreciating how the molecular level translates to function at the organ level). Most associated with the work of Ludwig von Bertalanffy.

Medical humanism: A model of medicine that combines biological reductionism about disease with a humanistic appreciation for the person who has the disease. Most associated with the work of William Osler. Its psychiatric application is found, in my view, in the work of Karl Jaspers. Contrasts with *biopsychosocial model.*

Metaphor: The use of a visual image or concrete object to signify the meaning of a word. It is believed that most, if not all, words have metaphors rooted in their etymology. In current usage, metaphors are contrasted with abstract language, which consists of imageless concepts such as good or truth. Mathematical symbols are pure abstractions

Method: The means by which psychiatric theories are derived. How we understand psychiatry. In psychoanalysis, for instance, the key method is free association. Multiple theories are derived from that method, but one understands those theories best by approaching them initially from what they share in common as a method. Based on Jaspers's dictum: "Between fact and method no sharp line can be drawn." Contrast with *theory.*

Method-based psychiatry: Focuses on methods, rather than content, believing that methods determine content. The right method should be used for the appropriate condition or illness. Contrast with *evidence-based medicine.* A synonym for *pluralism* (see below).

Pluralism: Also could be termed "method-based psychiatry." The view that certain methods are more correct than others for specific conditions or circumstances. Less is more. Use methods purely, combine them sequentially, not simultaneously. Only one theory or method is correct, but it is not the same for all aspects of psychiatry. Choice of method is based on empirical data if available and on conceptual soundness otherwise. One must justify one's choice of method conceptually or empirically; it is not a matter of mere preference. In political analogy: law-governed liberal democracy. See contrast with *eclecticism.*

Positivism: The view of science in which facts stand by themselves, separate from theories and methods. The view that inductive experience can lead to absolute truth. Contrast with *pragmatism, postmodernism,* and *pluralism.*

Postmodernism: The notion that there is no absolute truth, in science or medicine or psychiatry or politics. All human activity involves "discourses" that ultimately are based on power, not truth.

Pragmatism: As a philosophical school, based on the view that truth is not an abstract entity to which our ideas correspond; truth is appreciated by observing the results of our ideas in the real world of experience. Different pragmatic philosophies can be committed to the independent reality of truth (Charles Sanders Peirce) or deny such reality (William James, postmodernism). See *postmodernism.*

Science: The attempt to know truth based on testing hypotheses by experiment and experience. It can be positivistic or nonpositivistic. See *positivism.* Positivistic science is synonymous with biological *dogmatism* or *evidence-based medicine* or pure *Erklären.* Nonpositivistic science is synonymous with *pluralism* or *method-based psychiatry* or use of both *Erklären* and *Verstehen.*

Theory: The result of method.

Verstehen: Meaningful understanding. Associated with subjective, first-person knowledge. Attends to the uniquely individual aspects of phenomena. Focuses on the meaning of events or phenomena, as opposed to their causes. Contrasts with *Erklären.*

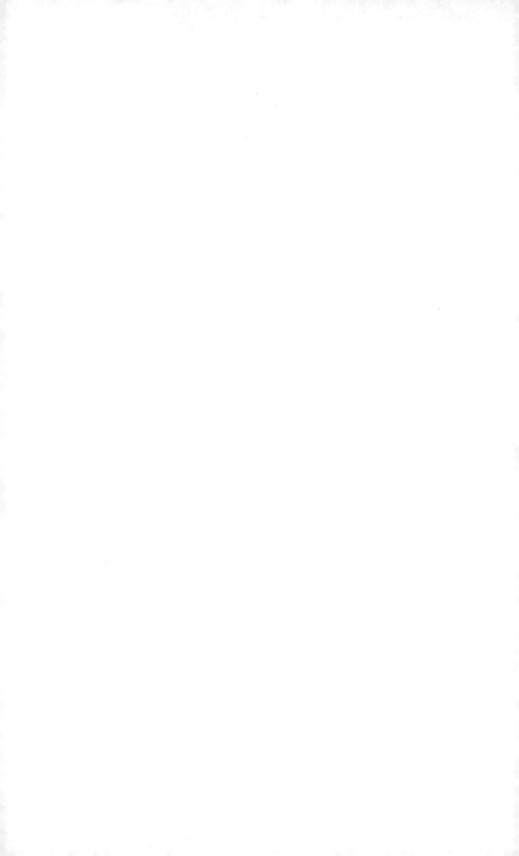

References

Abel, T. 1974. The operation called *Verstehen*. In Verstehen: *Subjective Understanding in the Social Sciences,* edited M. Truzzi. Reading, MA: Addison-Wesley Publishers.

Abramson, J. 2008. *Overdosed America.* New York: Harper.

Abroms, E. M. 1983. Beyond eclecticism. *Am J Psychiatry* 140(6):740–45.

Abroms, G. M. 1969. The new eclecticism. *Arch Gen Psychiatry* 20(5):514–23.

Ader, R., and A. H. Schmale Jr. 1980. George Libman Engel: On the occasion of his retirement. *Psychosom Med* 42 (1 Suppl):79–101.

American Psychiatric Association. 1980. *Diagnositic and Statistical Manual of Mental Disorders,* 3rd ed. Washington, DC: American Psychiatric Association.

Arieti, S, ed. 1974. *American Handbook of Psychiatry.* New York: Basic Books.

Austin, J. L. 1975. *How to Do Things with Words.* Cambridge, MA: Harvard University Press.

Baldessarini, R. J., S. N. Ghaemi, and A. C. Viguera. 2002. Tolerance in antidepressant treatment. *Psychother Psychosom* 71(4):177–79.

Barondess, J. A. 2002. Is Osler dead? *Perspect Biol Med* 45(1):65–84.

Bech, P. 2006. The full story of lithium: A tribute to Mogens Schou (1918–2005). *Psychother Psychosom* 75(5):265–69.

Beeson, P. B., and McDermott, W. 1971. *Cecil's Textbook of Medicine,* 13th ed. Philadelphia: Saunders.

Berkman, L. F., and Kawachi I. (Eds.) 2000. *Social Epidemiology.* New York: Oxford University Press.

Bliss, M. 1999. *William Osler: A Life in Medicine.* New York: Oxford University Press.

Bloom, A. 1988. *The Closing of the American Mind.* New York: Simon and Schuster.

Borges, J. L. 2000. *This Craft of Verse.* Cambridge, MA: Harvard University Press.

Borrell-Carrio, F., A. L. Suchman, and R. M. Epstein. 2004. The biopsychosocial model 25 years later: Principles, practice, and scientific inquiry. *Ann Fam Med* 2(6):576–82.

Bracken, P., and P. Thomas. 2001. Postpsychiatry: A new direction for mental health. *BMJ* 322(7288):724–27.

Breedlove, C. 1998. *Uncharted Lines.* Berkeley, CA: Ten Speed Press.

Brendel, D. 2006. *Healing Psychiatry.* Cambridge, MA: MIT Press.

Brown, T. M. 2000. The growth of George Engel's biopsychosocial model. Available from www.human-nature.com/free-associations.

———. 2003. George Engel and Rochester's biopsychosocial tradition: Historical and developmental perspectives. In *The Biopsychosocial Approach: Past, Present, Future,* edited by R. Frankel, T. Quill, and S. McDaniel. Rochester, NY: University of Rochester Press.

Burnham, J. C. 1983. *Jelliffe, American Psychoanalyst and Physician.* Chicago: University of Chicago Press.

Cade, J. F. 1949. Lithium salts in the treatment of psychotic excitement. *Med J Aust* 3 (Sept):349–52.

Campbell, W. H, and R. M. Rohrbaugh. 2006. *The Biopsychosocial Formulation Manual: A Guide for Mental Health Professionals.* New York: Routledge.

Cody, W. K. 1996. Drowning in eclecticism. *Nurs Sci Q* 9 (3):86–88.

Coles, R. 1989. *The Call of Stories.* Boston: Houghton-Mifflin.

Connor, J. T. 1991. "A sort of felo-de-se": Eclecticism, related medical sects, and their decline in Victorian Ontario. *Bull Hist Med* 65 (4):503–27.

Cotton, H. 1921. *The Defective, Delinquent, and Insane.* Princeton, NJ: Princeton University Press.

Dannefer, E. F., E. M. Hundert, and L. C. Henson. 2003. Medical education reform at the University of Rochester and the biopsychosocial tradition. In *The Biopsychosocial Approach: Past, Present, Future,* edited by R. Frankel, T. Quill, and S. McDaniel. Rochester, NY: University of Rochester Press.

Davey Smith, G. 2005. The biopsychosocial approach: A note of caution. In *Biopsychosocial Medicine: An Integrated Approach to Understanding Illness,* edited by P. White. Oxford: Oxford University Press.

Davidson, L., M. S. Lawless, and F. Leary. 2005. Concepts of recovery: Competing or complementary? *Curr Opin Psychiatry* 18(6):664–67.

deGruy, F. V. 2003. A biopsychosocial perspective on mental disorders: Depression in the primary care setting. In *The Biopsychosocial Approach: Past, Present, Future,* edited by R. Frankel, T. Quill, and S. McDaniel. Rochester, NY: University of Rochester Press.

Dennett, D. 1991. *Consciousness Explained.* Boston: Little, Brown, and Co.

———. 1995. *Darwin's Dangerous Idea.* New York: Simon and Schuster.

———. 1998. Postmodernism and truth. Available at http://ase.tufts.edu/cogstud/papers/postmod.tru.htm.

Dilthey, W. 1974. On the special character of the human sciences. In Verstehen: *Subjective Understanding in the Social Sciences,* edited by M. Truzzi. Reading, MA: Addison-Wesley Publishers.

———. 1985. *Poetry and Experience.* Edited by R. Makkreel and F. Rodi, *Selected Works,* vol. 5. Princeton, NJ: Princeton University Press.

Dimond, R. E., R. A. Havens, and A. C. Jones. 1978. A conceptual framework for the practice of prescriptive eclecticism in psychotherapy. *Am Psychol* 33(3):239–48.

Dombeck, M., K. Markakis, L. Brachman, B. Dalal, and T. Olsan. 2003. Analysis of a biopsychosocial correspondence: Models, mentors, and meanings. In *The Biopsychosocial Approach: Past, Present, Future,* edited by R. Frankel, T. Quill, and S. McDaniel. Rochester, NY: University of Rochester Press.

Double, D. 2002. The limits of psychiatry. *BMJ* 324(7342):900–904.

———. 2007. Adolf Meyer's psychobiology and the challenge for biomedicine. *Philos Psychiatr Psychol* 14:331–40.

Drossman, D. 2005. A case of irritable bowel syndrome that illustrates the biopsychosocial model of illness. In *Biopsychosocial Medicine: An Integrated Approach to Understanding Illness,* edited by P. White. Oxford: Oxford University Press.

Drury, S. B. 1994. *Alexandre Kojeve: The Roots of Postmodern Politics.* New York: Macmillan.

Eastman, M. 1921. *Enjoyment of Poetry.* New York: C. Scribner's Sons.

Einstein, A. 1950. *Out of My Later Years.* New York: Philosophical Library.

El-Hai, J. 2005. *The Lobotomist.* New York: Wiley.

Engel, G. L. 1960. A unified concept of health and disease. *Perspect Biol Med* 3:459–85.

———. 1967. The concept of psychosomatic disorder. *J Psychosom Res* 11(1):3–9.

———. 1977. The need for a new medical model: a challenge for biomedicine. *Science* 196(4286):129–36.

———. 1978. The biopsychosocial model and the education of health professionals. *Ann N Y Acad Sci* 310:169–87.

———. 1980. The clinical application of the biopsychosocial model. *Am J Psychiatry* 137:535–44.

———. 1987. Physician-scientists and scientific physicians: Resolving the humanism-science dichotomy. *Am J Med* 82:107–11.

———. 1992. How much longer must medicine's science be bound by a seventeenth-century world view? *Psychother Psychosom* 57 (1–2):3–16.

Engel, P. A. 2001. George L. Engel, M.D., 1913–1999: Remembering his life and work; rediscovering his soul. *Psychosomatics* 42(2):94–99.

Engstrom, E. 2004. *Clinical Psychiatry in Imperial Germany.* Ithaca, NY: Cornell University Press.

Epstein, R. M., D. S. Morse, G. C. Williams, P. LeRoux, A. L. Suchman, and T. E. Quill. 2003. Clinical practice and the biopsychosocial approach. In *The Biopsychosocial Approach: Past, Present, Future,* edited by R. Frankel, T. Quill, and S. McDaniel. Rochester, NY: University of Rochester Press.

Ermarth, M. 1978. *Wilhelm Dilthey: The Critique of Historical Reason.* Chicago: University of Chicago Press.

Evans, J. G. 1995. Evidence-based and evidence-biased medicine. *Age Ageing* 24(6):461–63.

Eysenck, H. J. 1952. The effects of psychotherapy: An evaluation. *J Consult Clin Psychol* 16:319–24.

Fava, G. A. 1992. The concept of psychosomatic disorder. *Psychother Psychosom* 58(1): 1–12.

———. 2000. On looking inward and being scientific: A tribute to GL Engel MD. *Psychother Psychosom* 69:169.

———. 2006. A different medicine is possible. *Psychother Psychosom* 75(1):1–3.

Fava, G. A., and N. Sonino. 2005. The clinical domains of psychosomatic medicine. *J Clin Psychiatry* 66(7):849–58.

Feynman, R. 1988. *What Do You Care What Other People Think?* New York: Bantam.

Foucault, M. 1988. *Madness and Civilization.* New York: Vintage.

Frank, E., D. J. Kupfer, J. M. Perel, C. Cornes, D. B. Jarrett, A. G. Mallinger, M. E. Thase, A. B. McEachran, and V. J. Grochocinski. 1990. Three-year outcomes for maintenance therapies in recurrent depression. *Arch Gen Psychiatry* 47:1093–99.

Frank, J. D., and J. B. Frank 1991. *Persuasion and Healing: A Comparative Study of Psychotherapy,* 3rd ed. Baltimore: Johns Hopkins University Press.

Frankel, R. M., T. E. Quill, and S. H. McDaniel, eds. 2003. *The Biopsychosocial Approach: Past, Present, Future.* Rochester, NY: University of Rochester Press.

Frankfurt, H. G. 2005. *On Bullshit*. Princeton, NJ: Princeton University Press.

Frankl, V. E. 1955/1986. *The Doctor and the Soul*. New York: Vintage.

Fulford, B., T. Thornton, and G. Graham. 2006. *Oxford Textbook of Philosophy and Psychiatry*. New York: Oxford University Press.

Fulford, K. W. M. 1989. *Moral Theory and Medical Practice*. Cambridge: Cambridge University Press.

Fulford, K. W. M., M. Broome, G. Stanghellini, and T. Thornton. 2005. Looking with both eyes open: Fact and value in psychiatric diagnosis? *World Psychiatry* 4(2):78–86.

Gabbard, G. O., and J. Kay. 2001. The fate of integrated treatment: Whatever happened to the biopsychosocial psychiatrist? *Am J Psychiatry* 158(12):1956–63.

Galbraith, J. K. 1958. *The Affluent Society*. Boston: Houghton Mifflin.

Garfield, S. L., and R. Kurtz. 1977. A study of eclectic views. *J Consult Clin Psychol* 45(1):78–83.

Geppert, C. 2008. Why psychiatrists should read the humanities. *Psychiatric Times* 2.

Gerth, H., and C. W. Mills, eds. 1948. *From Max Weber: Essays in Sociology*. New York: Taylor & Francis.

Ghaemi, S. N. 1999. Performative statements and the will: Mechanisms of psychotherapeutic change. *Am J Psychother* 53(4):483–94.

———. 2003. *The Concepts of Psychiatry: A Pluralistic Approach to the Mind and Mental Illness*. Baltimore: Johns Hopkins University Press.

———. 2007. Adolf Meyer: Psychiatric anarchist. *Philos Psychiatr Psychol* 14:341–46.

———. 2008. Toward a Hippocratic psychopharmacology. *Can J Psychiatry* 53(3):189–96.

Goin, M. K. 2005. A current perspective on the psychotherapies. *Psychiatr Serv* 56(3):255–57.

Goldstein, S. G., R. E. Deysack, and R. A. Kleinknecht. 1973. Effect of experience and amount of information on identification of cerebral impairment. *J Consult Clin Psychol* 41:330–34.

Grinker, R. R., Jr. 1994. Remarks at the presentation of the Presidential Award for Distinguished Service and Scientific Contributions to Roy R. Grinker, Sr., M.D. *J Am Acad Psychoanal* 22(2):321–29.

Grinker, R. R., Sr. 1964a. Psychiatry rides madly in all directions. *Arch Gen Psychiatry* 10:228–37.

———. 1964b. A struggle for eclecticism. *Am J Psychiatry* 121:451–57.

———. 1965. The sciences of psychiatry: Fields, fences and riders. *Am J Psychiatry* 122(4):367–76.

———. 1966. "Open-system" psychiatry. *Am J Psychoanal* 26(2):115–28.

———. 1969. An essay on schizophrenia and science. *Arch Gen Psychiatry* 20(1):1–24.

———. 1970. The continuing search for meaning. *Am J Psychiatry* 127(6):725–31.

———. 1975. The future educational needs of psychiatrists. *Am J Psychiatry* 132(3):259–62.

———. 1976. In memory of Ludwig von Bertalanffy's contribution to psychiatry. *Behav Sci* 21(4):207–18.

———. 1977. Twenty years of psychoanalysis: Retrospect and prospect. *J Am Acad Psychoanal* 5(1):79–93.

————. 1994. Training of a psychiatrist-psychoanalyst. *J Am Acad Psychoanal* 22(2): 343–50.

Hall, G. S., and S. Freud. 1960. Sigmund Freud and G. Stanley Hall: Exchange of letters. *Psychoanalytic Q* 29:307–16.

Hammad, T. A., T. Laughren, and J. Racoosin. 2006. Suicidality in pediatric patients treated with antidepressant drugs. *Arch Gen Psychiatry* 63(3):332–39.

Havens, L. L. 1967. Karl Jaspers and American psychiatry. *Am J Psychiatry* 124(1):66–70.

————. 1984. The need for tests of normal functioning in the psychiatric interview. *Am J Psychiatry* 141(10):1208–11.

————. 1985a. Historical perspectives on diagnosis in psychiatry. *Compr Psychiatry* 26(4):326–36.

————. 1985b. *Participant Obsevation*. Montvale, NJ: Jason Aronson.

————. 1986. *Making Contact: Uses of Language in Psychotherapy*. Cambridge, MA: Harvard University Press.

————. 1987. *Approaches to the Mind: Movement of the Psychiatric Schools from Sects toward Science*. Cambridge, MA: Harvard University Press. (Original publication in 1973)

————. 1993. *Coming to Life: Reflections on the Art of Psychotherapy*. Cambridge, MA: Harvard University Press.

————. 1994. The performative function of psychotherapy. Unpublished manuscript.

————. 1996. *A Safe Place: Laying the Groundwork for Psychotherapy*. Cambridge, MA: Harvard University Press.

————. 2005. *Psychiatric Movements*. Piscataway, NJ: Transaction Publishers, Rutgers University Press.

Healy, D. 1998. *The Antidepressant Era*. Cambridge, MA: Harvard University Press.

————. 2001. *The Creation of Psychopharmacology*. Cambridge, MA: Harvard University Press.

————. 2006. The latest mania: Selling bipolar disorder. *PLoS Med* 3(4):e185.

————. 2008. *Mania: A Brief History of Bipolar Disorder*. Baltimore: Johns Hopkins University Press.

Hempel, C. G. 1965. *Aspects of Scientific Explanation*. New York: Free Press.

Jaspers, K. 1989. *On Max Weber*. New York: Paragon House.

————. 1997 (1959). *General Psychopathology*, translated by J. Hoenig and M. Hamilton. 2 vols. Baltimore: Johns Hopkins University Press.

Jouanna, J. 1999. *Hippocrates*. Baltimore: Johns Hopkins University Press.

Kandel, E. R. 1998. A new intellectual framework for psychiatry. *Am J Psychiatry* 155: 457–69.

Kavka, J. 1999. *The Analytic Observer: Newsletter of the Chicago Psychoanalytic Society* 7, no. 1 (March 1999) [retrieved February 24, 2007]. Available from www.3b.com/cps/newsletters/1999/03/index.htm#Institute/Society%20Archives.

Kendler, K. S. 1990. Toward a scientific psychiatric nosology. *Arch Gen Psychiatry* 47: 969–73.

————. 2005. Toward a philosophical structure for psychiatry. *Am J Psychiatry* 162 (3): 433–40.

Kety, S. S. 1960. A biologist examines the mind and behavior. *Science* 132:1861–67.

Kleijnen, J. 2005. How important is the biopsychosocial approach? Some examples from research. In *Biopsychosocial Medicine: An Integrated Approach to Understanding Illness,* edited by P. White. Oxford: Oxford University Press.

Klerman, G. L. 1986. Historical perspectives on contemporary schools of psychopathology. In *Contempory Directions in Psychopathology: Toward the* DSM-IV, edited by T. Millon and G. Klerman. New York: Guilford Press.

Kojeve, A. 1980. *Introduction to the Reading of Hegel.* Ithaca, NY: Cornell University Press.

Kuhn, T. 1962/1996. *The Structure of Scientific Revolutions.* Chicago: University of Chicago Press.

Kushner, H. I. 1998. Beyond social construction: Toward new histories of psychiatry. *J History of the Neurosciences* 7:141–49.

Kushner, H. I., and Sterk, C. E. 2005. The limits of social capital: Durkeim, suicide, and social cohesion. *Am J Public Health* 95: 1139–43

Kushner, H. I. 2006. Taking biology seriously: The next task for historians of addiction? *Bull Hist Med* 80: 115–43

Laing, R. D. 1969. *The Divided Self.* Baltimore: Pelican.

Lakoff, G, and M Johnson. 1980. *Metaphors We Live By.* Chicago: University of Chicago Press.

Lazarus, A. A. 1990. Can psychotherapists transcend the shackles of their training and superstitions? *J Clin Psychol* 46(3):351–58.

Leopardi, G. 1983. *Moral Tales.* Manchester, UK: Carcanet Press.

Lewis, A. 1967. *The State of Psychiatry: Essays and Addresses.* New York: Science House.

Lewis, B. 2006. *Moving beyond Prozac, DSM, and the New Psychiatry.* Ann Arbor: University of Michigan Press.

———. 2007. The biopsychosocial model and philosophic pragmatism: Is George Engel a pragmatist? *Philos Psychiatr Psychol* 14:299–310.

Mack, J. E. 2007. *Abduction: Human Encounters with Aliens.* New York: Scribner.

Macklin, R. 1973. The medical model in psychoanalysis and psychotherapy. *Compr Psychiatry* 14(1):49–69.

Makkreel, R., ed. 1991. *Wilhelm Dilthey: Selected Works,* vol. 1. Princeton, NJ: Princeton University Press.

———. 1992. *Dilthey: Philosopher of the Human Studies.* Princeton, NJ: Princeton University Press.

Malmgren, H. 2005. The theoretical basis of the biopsychosocial model. In *Biopsychosocial Medicine: An Integrated Approach to Understanding Illness,* edited by P. White. Oxford: Oxford University Press.

Marguelis, A. M. 1989. *The Empathic Imagination.* New York: Norton.

Markowitz, J. C. 2005. Psychotherapy and eclecticism. *Psychiatr Serv* 56(5):612.

Marmot, M. 2005. Remediable or preventable social factors in the aetiology and prognosis of medical disorders. In *Biopsychosocial Medicine: An Integrated Approach to Understanding Illness,* edited by P. White. Oxford: Oxford University Press.

McHugh, P. R. 1987. William Osler and the new psychiatry. *Ann Intern Med* 107(6):914–18.

———. 2006. *The Mind Has Mountains.* Baltimore: Johns Hopkins University Press.

McHugh, P. R., and P. R. Slavney. 1998. *The Perspectives of Psychiatry.* Baltimore: Johns Hopkins University Press. (Originally published in 1983)

McIntosh, D. 1977. The objective bases of Max Weber's ideal types. *History and Theory* 16:265–79.

McLaren, N. 1998. A critical review of the biopsychosocial model. *Aust N Z J Psychiatry* 32:86–92.

Menand, L. 2002. *The Metaphysical Club*. New York: Farrar, Strauss, and Giroux.

Mencken, HL. 1982. *Mencken Chrestomathy*. New York: Vintage.

Meyer, A. 1948. *The Commonsense Psychiatry of Adolf Meyer*. New York: McGraw Hill.

Moncrieff, J. 2006. Psychiatric drug promotion and the politics of neo-liberalism. *Br J Psychiatry* 188:301–2.

Muir, L. J., and G. Muir. 1937. *Muir's Thesaurus of Truths*. Salt Lake City, UT: Deseret News Press.

Muller, R. J. 2008. *Doing Psychiatry Wrong*. New York: Analytic Press.

Muncie, W. S. 1974. The psychobiological approach. In *American Handbook of Psychiatry*, vol. 1, edited by S. Arieti. New York: Basic Books.

Nagel, E. 1953. On the method of *Verstehen* as the sole method of philosophy. *J Philos* 50:154–57.

Norcross, J. C., C. P. Karpiak, and K. M. Lister. 2005. What's an integrationist? A study of self-identified integrative and (occasionally) eclectic psychologists. *J Clin Psychol* 61(12):1587–94.

Nussbaum, M. 1996. *The Therapy of Desire*. Princeton, NJ: Princeton University Press.

Oakes, G. 1988. *Weber and Rickert*. Cambridge, MA: MIT Press.

Odegaard, C. 1986. *Dear Doctor: A Personal Letter to a Physician*. Menlo Park, NJ: Henry J. Kaiser Family Foundation.

Okasha, S. 2002. *Philosophy of Science: A Very Short Introduction*. New York: Oxford University Press.

Osler, W. 1948. *Aequanimitas*. Philadelphia: Blakiston Co.

Pies, R. W. 2007, Sept 25. Metaphor and meaning: How words work magic in our patients. *Yale J Humanities Med*. Available at http://yjhm.yale.edu/essays/rpies2007 0925.htm.

Pinel, P. 1983. *A Treatise on Insanity*, translated by D. Davis. Birmingham, AL: Classics of Medicine Library. (Originally published in 1806)

Popper, K. 1959. *The Logic of Scientific Discovery*. New York: Basic Books.

Reiser, M. F. 1980. Implications of a biopsychosocial model for research in psychiatry. *Psychosom Med* 42(1 Suppl):141–51.

Rickman, H. P. 1988. *Dilthey Today*. New York: Greenwood Press.

Roazen, P. 1993a. *Canada's King: An Essay in Political Psychology*. New York: Mosaic Press.

———. 1993b. *Freud and His Followers*. New York: New York University Press.

Robins, E., and S. B. Guze. 1970. Establishment of diagnostic validity in psychiatric illness: its application to schizophrenia. *Am J Psychiatry* 126:983–87.

Ros-Janet, J. G. 2005. *Del Conocimiento Poetico* (Of Poetic Knowledge). Panama City, Panama: Imprenta Articsa.

Sackett, D. L., S. Strauss, W. S. Richardson, W. Rosenberg, and R. B. Haynes. 2000. *Evidence Based Medicine*, 2nd ed. London: Churchill Livingstone.

Sadler, J. Z., and Y. F. Hulgus. 1992. Clinical problem solving and the biopsychosocial model. *Am J Psychiatry* 149(10):1315–23.

Santayana, G. 1924. *Character and Opinion in the United States.* New York: C. Scribner's Sons.

Schou, M., N. Juel-Nielsen, E. Stromgren, and H. Voldby. 1954. The treatment of manic psychosis by the administration of lithium salts. *J Neurol Psychiatry* 17:250–60.

Schwartz, M. A., and O. P. Wiggins. 1986. Logical empiricism and psychiatric classification. *Comprehensive Psychiatry* 27:101–14.

———. 1987. Diagnosis and ideal types. *Comprehensive Psychiatry* 28:277–291.

Sharfstein, S. S. 2005. Recovery movement will strengthen psychiatrist-patient relationship. (http://pn.psychiatryonline.org/cgi/content/full/40/20/3).

Shay, J. 1995. *Achilles in Vietnam.* New York: Simon and Schuster.

Shorter, E. 2005. The history of the biopsychosocial approach in medicine: Before and after Engel. In *Biopsychosocial Medicine: An Integrated Approach to Understanding Illness,* edited by P. White. Oxford: Oxford University Press.

Simon, R. M. 1974. On eclecticism. *Am J Psychiatry* 131(2):135–39.

Slavney, P. R., and P. R. McHugh. 1987. *Psychiatric Polarities.* Baltimore: Johns Hopkins University Press.

Snow, C. P. 1993. *The Two Cultures.* Cambridge: Cambridge University Press. (Lectures originally given in 1959)

Soldani, F., S. N. Ghaemi, and R. J. Baldessarini. 2005. Research reports on treatments for bipolar disorder: Preliminary assessment of methodological quality. *Acta Psychiatr Scand* 112(1):72–74.

Sontag, S. 1978. *Illness as Metaphor.* New York: Farrar, Strauss, and Giroux.

Sowers, W. 2005. Transforming systems of care: the American Association of Community Psychiatrists Guidelines for Recovery Oriented Services. *Community Ment Health J* 41(6):757–74.

Stigler, S. M. 1986. *The History of Statistics.* Cambridge, MA: Harvard University Press.

Stock, S. L., G. Catalano, J. D. Dreier, M. M. Ross, and M. C. Catalano. 2006. A survey of psychiatry residency programs: Association between program characteristics and success in the 2003 NRMP. *Psychiatr Q* 77(4):293–305.

Stone, A. A. 1981. Psychiatrists and eclecticism. *Am J Psychiatry* 138(2):257–58.

Szasz, T. S. 1970. *Ideology and Insanity.* New York: Doubleday.

———. 1984. *The Myth of Mental Illness.* New York: Harper. (Originally published 1960)

Thase, M. E. 1997. Psychotherapy of refractory depressions. *Depress Anxiety* 5(4):190–201.

Trimble, M. R. 2007. *The Soul in the Brain: The Cerebral Basis of Language, Art, and Belief.* Baltimore: Johns Hopkins University Press.

Truzzi, M., ed. 1974. *Verstehen: Subjective Understanding in the Social Sciences.* Reading, MA: Addison-Wesley Publishers.

Tucker, W. T. 1965. Max Weber's "*Verstehen.*" *Sociol Q* 6:157–65.

van Praag, H. M. 1980. Tablets and talking: A spurious contrast in psychiatry. *Comprehensive Psychiatry* 20:502–10.

von Bertalanffy, L. 1974. General system theory and psychiatry. In *American Handbook of Psychiatry,* edited by S. Arieti. New York: Basic Books.

Von Wright, G. H. 1971. *Explanation and Understanding.* Ithaca, NY: Cornell University Press.

Weber, M. 1974. On subjective interpretation in the social sciences. In Verstehen: *Subjective Understanding in the Social Sciences*, edited by M. Truzzi. Reading, MA: Addison-Wesley Publishers.

Wessely, S. 2005. Foreword. In *Biopsychosocial Medicine: An Integrated Approach to Understanding Illness*, edited by P. White. Oxford: Oxford University Press.

White, P., ed. 2005. *Biopsychosocial Medicine: An Integrated Approach to Understanding Illness*. Oxford: Oxford University Press.

Wiggins, O. P., and M. A. Schwartz. 1991. Is there a science of meaning? *Integrative Psychiatry* 7:48–53.

———. 1997. Edmund Husserl's influence on Karl Jaspers' phenomenology. *Philos Psychiatr Psychol* 4:15–36.

Williams, D. C. 1954. The new eclecticism. *Can J Psychol* 8(3):113–24.

Williams, G. C., R. M. Frankel, T. L. Campbell, and E. L. Deci. 2003. The science of the art of medicine: Research on the biopsychosocial approach to health care. In *The Biopsychosocial Approach: Past, Present, Future*, edited by R. Frankel, T. Quill, and S. McDaniel. Rochester, NY: University of Rochester Press.

Williams, W. C. 1983. *Selected Poems*. Coney Island, NY: New Directions Publishing.

Wilson, E. O. 1998. *Consilience*. New York: Random House.

Wynne, L. C. 2003. Systems theory and the biopsychosocial approach. In *The Biopsychosocial Approach: Past, Present, Future*, edited by R. Frankel, T. Quill, and S. McDaniel. Rochester, NY: University of Rochester Press.

Yager, J. 1977. Psychiatric eclecticism: a cognitive view. *Am J Psychiatry* 134(7):736–41.

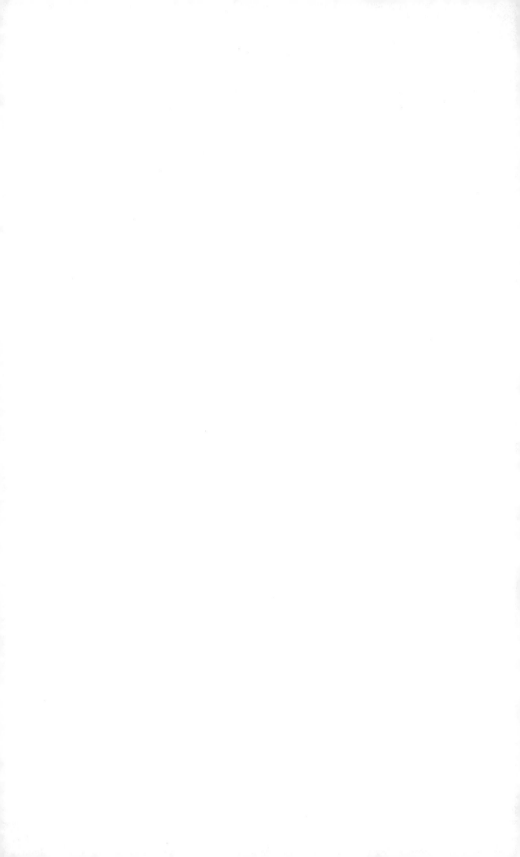

Index

abstraction, 152–53, 172, 179–81, 203–4

antidepressants, 49, 72–73, 105–6, 109–11, 195

anxiety, 36, 49, 74, 105, 214, 227n1

art(s), 134, 143, 155, 163, 165, 193; medicine, 25, 92, 96, 140–41, 209; science, 87–88, 133

behaviorism: BPS model, 36, 105, 138–39; criticism, 22–23, 67, 84, 88; knowledge, 65, 162–63, 180, 184–85, 192–95; in practice, 12–15, 43, 54, 117

biological component, mental illness, 4, 62, 110; Engel, 42–43, 82, 227n1; Grinker, 23, 34–36; postmodern, 116–17, 124, 135–38, 206–7, 210, 214

biological reductionism, 22, 100–101, 124, 209, 213–14, 234; Engel, 43, 45, 50, 224n3, 225n4, 229n2; Osler, 130–31, 143–44

biomedicine, 93, 134, 192–95; dehumanized, 92, 119, 128, 137, 198, 208; reductionism, 4–5, 33, 47, 58–60; views on, 43–45, 96, 101, 129, 141, 210

biopsychosocial (BPS) model, 119, 233; central aspect, 44, 62–63, 132–33; combination therapy, 113–14; criticism, 81–83, 116–17, 189, 211–15; dogmatism, 112–13, 133–34; doubts, ix–x, 13, 56, 76–77, 94, 123, 198; EBM replacement, 123–27; eclecticism, 16–17, 81, 117, 164, 213–14; emptiness, 192–94; Engel, 5, 25, 27, 33–50, 53, 133–34, 217, 223n3–225n4; Grinker, 5, 32–35, 51, 53, 85, 222n2, 223nn3–4; humanism, 60–63, 82, 95–96, 128, 135–37, 209–10; label, 35, 42, 212, 215, 223n4; Meyer, 3–7, 10, 27, 65, 67; new/old, 12–14, 124, 211–12; pharmacology vs., 103–4, 108–11; philosophy, 57–58, 226n4; pluralism, 194–95; policy making, 84–85; psychoanalysis vs., 63–64, 82, 133, 137–40; psychosomatic application, 53–56; psychotherapy need, 74–75, 98–99; pub-

lic health, 58–60; research blueprint, 45, 81–89, 114, 227n1; science/humanities, 47–49, 159–66, 230n6; teaching, 62, 91–94, 101, 217, 227n1, 228n2; validity, 56–62, 88, 226n2; *Verstehen* vs., 163–64, 167

BPS. *See* biopsychosocial model

cardiovascular disease, 46–47, 60, 63, 142, 214

causality: explanation, 164–65, 173–74, 177–80, 183; illness, 4–5, 53–56, 59, 134

clinical diagnosis, 129–30, 189, 195–96; criteria, 70–71, 73–77, 205–8; pharmacology, 104–5, 109–11; science, 70, 85, 106–7, 224n3

clinical interview/history, 95–96, 129, 131, 134–35, 190

clinical skills, teaching, 129–31, 134–35, 142–44

clinical trials, 71–72, 88, 125

clinicopathological method, 39, 129–30

cognitive process, 105, 133, 160, 163; BPS model, 137–39; eclecticism, 16, 20–21; intellect, 154–57, 202, 220; meaning, 97, 150, 169–78, 191

cognitive therapies, 14, 84, 88, 165

colectomy, 7–10

collaboration, 93, 100–101, 109, 125, 208

combination therapy, 53–54, 63–64, 74–75, 103, 107, 113–16, 226n3

communication, 23, 25, 93, 96–97, 172, 190; types/modes, 149, 156–57, 184–86, 208

conceptual context: BPS model, 5, 23, 95, 228n2; disease, 222n3; of EBM, 126–27; eclecticism, 12–21, 25–26, 186; health, 4–5, 88, 107–10, 124, 192, 201–2, 208, 224n3; ideal experiences, 169, 180–81, 193; psychotherapy, 114, 118–19; residencies, 218–19

consciousness, 182, 189, 199, 204, 212

coping mechanisms, 43, 138–39, 224n3